THIRD PARTY RAPE

The Conspiracy to Rob You of Health Care

C. Norman Shealy, M.D., Ph.D.

1993
Galde Press
St. Paul, Minnesota

FIRST EDITION

Library of Congress Cataloging-in-Publication Data

Shealy, C. Norman, 1932–
    Third party rape : the conspiracy to rob you of health care /
C. Norman Shealy
        p.   cm.
    Includes bibliographical references.
    ISBN 1–880090–07–4 : $12.95
    1. Medical care—Cost control.   2. Insurance. Health—Cost
control.   3. Health behavior.   4. Medical care—United States—Cost
control.   5. Insurance, Health—United States—Cost control.
I. Title.
RA410.5.S42   1993
362.1—dc20   93-7684
                                                                      CIP

 Printed on recycled paper.

The opinions expressed in this book are not necessarily those of the publisher.

Galde Press, Inc.
P.O. Box 65611
St. Paul, Minnesota 55165

Acknowledgments

I have collected information and articles for this book since 1970. During the writing many friends have contributed specific anecdotes and numerous additional documents. For chapters 5 and 6 I received considerable legal assistance.

I particularly acknowledge my partner, Dr. Roger Cady, who has assumed responsibility for our clinic in order for me to retire prematurely and to be "free at last." My wife, Mary-Charlotte, and my friend, Caroline Myss, have made many useful editorial comments.

Julie Dennison has, as usual for her, done a herculean job organizing, typing, and retyping the manuscript. And I am indebted to Susan Robards for assistance in organizing the ongoing supportive documentation to back the startling facts presented in this book.

I also want to acknowledge the *exceptions* to the Third Party Mafia. There are some honest insurance companies, hospitals, and federal officials. And there are many lawyers who are not the "ambulance chasers" who give their profession a bad name. Unfortunately it is the majority of those who make up the Third Party who have created the chaos which we now face as a nation. To them I owe thanks for motivating me, with their shenanigans, to address these issues frankly and honestly as I see them.

Other Books by the Author

The Creation of Health with Caroline M. Myss

AIDS: Passageway to Transformation with Caroline M. Myss

Biogenics® Health Maintenance

Speedy Gourmet

To Parent or Not? with Mary-Charlotte Shealy

90 Days to Self-Health

The Pain Game

Occult Medicine Can Save Your Life with Arthur S. Freese

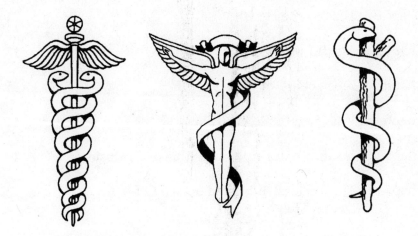

At left is the symbol of the caduceus, commonly understood to be a symbol of the medical profession. However, since it is the device normally carried by Mercury, god of thieves, it is an appropriate symbol for the Disease Insurance industry. The true symbol of medicine is not that of Hermes, but of Aesclepius, the fabled Greek physician. This symbol, shown at far right, features but one snake. The symbol in the center is that of chiropractic.

Table of Contents

Third Party Rape: A Philosophical Overview   ix

Chapter 1: Uniting the Health Wise   1

Chapter 2: The ILL-egalization of America   17

Chapter 3: Free at Last   35

Chapter 4: Who Gets Sick? Who Should Pay?   41

Chapter 5: Insurance Principles: An Area of Confusion   49

Chapter 6: The Doctors: Educated & Well-Off—
            Or Are They?   67

Chapter 7: To Pay Or Not to Pay?   77

Chapter 8: The Roots of Health   93

Chapter 9: The Stress Connection   107

Chapter 10: Reuniting Body, Mind, and Emotions
             With Spirit   145

Epilogue: A Case in Point   153

Annotated Bibliography   157

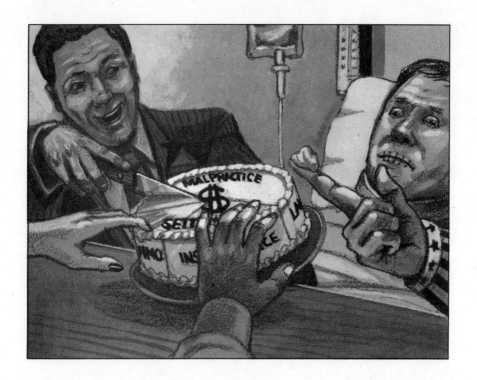

A Philosophical Overview

In the beginning there was Blue Cross/Blue Shield, which begat the "Evil Empire." Do you think I am exaggerating? Have you tried to use your health insurance recently? Since when does any company insure health? Indeed, it doesn't even insure the cost of being ill today.

My own emotional reactions to the Armageddon of today's medical insurance crisis will come through in this introductory chapter. However, as much as is humanly possible, I will furnish you the facts that support my reactions. Actually, I have been building files on the Third Party menace for at least 15 years. And, as you will see, the problem has been building since at least 1965, when the greatest fraud in the history of government was created: Medicare.

At the beginning, let me give you my most important bit of advice: Live the healthiest possible lifestyle and take out a $5,000 deductible major medical or catastrophic insurance. Invest $5,000 in a good money market and every year that you don't use any of the money for medical treatment, give yourself a bonus. Or leave the investment to grow to be used only for a major essential need.

Now let's look at some fascinating history. At the beginning of this century the average life expectancy was roughly half what it is now. But about 90% of the improvement in longevity comes in the *first 20 years of life*. In other words, the great advances have been in decreasing childhood death from infectious diseases. What about antibiotics? The evidence is overwhelming that the major improvements have been in sewage disposal, chlorination of water, pasteurization of milk, and provision of adequate calories. In fact, Dr. Thomas McEown has estimated that about 92% of increased longevity comes from these simple public health measures.

Who needs medical care? Mainly those with unhealthy lifestyles. Cigarette smoking; excess alcohol; obesity; failure to exercise; excess fat, salt and sugar; and failure to use seat belts or obey the speed limit account for about 75% of all illness and death! Take away those unhealthy lifestyle choices and you cut your chances of needing medical care by 75%. Add a few more specific habits and you probably can cut your risks of needing the system by 90% or more. Later I will outline for you the most optimal life path you can follow in order to avoid needing medical care.

Let us begin at the beginning. Until the late 1920s there was no medical insurance. Two hospitals in Texas then offered a policy for $6.00 per year, guaranteeing 20 days in hospital, mostly for surgery or obviously serious illness. The idea was as popular as communism to the John Birch Society! But it gradually spread, and about 10 years later the first insurance offering coverage for physician treatment, in hospital, mostly surgery, was introduced in Oregon. Physicians who participated were threatened with censure by the state medical society, and some lost their licenses. But by the early 1940s medical insurance began to be a desirable benefit and unions began demanding coverage. Nevertheless, medical insurance at that time was much like Social Security, a safety net to cover only some services in hospital. This fact alone explains why most insurance and most physician care has been strongly tilted, financially, toward surgeons, who make 2–10 times as much for their services as do general physicians.

By 1945 President Harry S. Truman was arguing that we spent only 4.5% of gross national product on "health" care; surely we could do more. And more we did, but not until 20 years later when Johnson ushered in the Great Society, which may have been the single greatest contributor to the crisis in medical costs. Unable to get national medical insurance past the AMA, the American Bar Association, farmers, and Congress, Truman settled for the Hill-Burton Act, which essentially doubled the number of hospitals and medical school graduates. Pressures from many fronts pushed for ever-increasing medical insurance, about 80% issued by the "Godfather," Blue Cross/Blue Shield, strongly hospitalization oriented. In 1967, I did a survey at one of the finest hospitals in the country. Over two-thirds of the patients in hospital were there not because they were sick enough to need hospitalization, but to get their insurance to cover. This illogical and cost-increasing restriction of medical insurance paved the way for bankrupting by Medicare. Introduced in 1965, Medicare led to a revolution in medical care. It, too, emphasized hospitalization and much higher pay for surgery. It also began the push to cover everything from medication to home care. Nursing homes became profitable, and soon our elderly, who had remained in the family, were warehoused. Home health services became profitable; life insurance companies that had had very little medical insurance pushed one another over at the government trough, vying for a growing piece of the action. Non-Medicare medical insurance grew, too, as greed on the part of the insurance industry was fueled by equal greed on the part of hospitals and nursing homes, with the active complicity of the medical profession. Within five years national headlines proclaimed a crisis in medical costs, as medical expenditures had tripled!

Since that time the Evil Empire has blamed physicians for rising and ever-escalating costs. But physician costs represent only 19% of medical costs. Hospitals cost over twice as much (39%), and nursing homes cost 8%. Home health care, drugs, and other medical products cost well above physician costs. Indeed, if physician costs were cut in half, an apparent goal of the "health" insurance industry and the federal government, working in cahoots, as the insurance industry is now the CIA and FBI for medical control, even then total medical costs would go down only 9.5%. Medical costs would still cost 10% or more of gross national product.

The Third Party also blames pharmaceuticals for "excessive" costs. But drug costs are significantly below those of lawyers, hospitals, insurance, nursing homes, etc. And, as with physicians, government regulations have markedly accelerated the costs of producing an approved drug.

In the early 1980s, in an attempt to cut Medicare costs, the government, with their henchmen, the insurance industry, introduced DRGs, one of the more illogical thoughts of the century. This has led to the bankruptcy of many hospitals; and apparently the goal is to close at least 25% of all hospitals. Meanwhile, the Evil Empire seized upon their new role as prosecutor of physicians and added patients as well. They embarked upon a system which has multiplied paper work, duplication, delay, and harassment, which is forcing many physicians to quit practice years before they would have done so ordinarily. There is a crescendo effect, leading to near chaos. Massachusetts passed a law that physicians had to accept Medicare assignment, automatically cutting their fees 30% or more. As a result, 40% of family physicians have left the state of Massachusetts. Increasing numbers of physicians refuse to see Medicare patients.

Medicaid is an even greater mess. States vary tremendously in what they pay for the care of the indigent, from 15% to 80% of usual fees. It is highly unlikely that any physician will remain in practice if fees are cut 85%! Actually that would bring physicians well below the national average, and physicians work, on average, 60 hours per week, 50% more than the average worker.

If you think I am overstating the problem, read an article from *The New England Journal of Medicine,* July 1990, "Health Care Rationing Through Inconvenience: The Third Party's Secret Weapon." For our most prestigious journal, that's strong stuff. Just the day I am writing this, actually using a word processor for the first time, a physician friend told me that he expects to walk away from his practice within two years, making his living from a multi-level marketing product. He said that he does not know a single physician his age who is not looking for a way to escape the Evil Empire.

You may have noticed by now that I do not use the term "Health Insurance." The reason is simple; there is no company offering even a token of real insurance to promote health. You may ask, "How about HMOs, Health Maintenance Organizations?" These, in general, are prepaid disease treatment organizations, begun in World War II by the Kaiser Corporation to control medical costs. And control they did! As late as the 1960s, Kaiser-Permante in California tried to get their neurosurgeons to diagnose malignant brain tumors as strokes, to avoid operating on them and to save money. Virtually all their neurosurgeons quit. Interestingly, it really would not have made much difference in ultimate outcome; but the principle is reprehensible! HMOs traditionally have been much less prone to push needless hospitalization; in fact, they discourage hospitalization. But they provide minimal health maintenance. If you are ill they provide medical treatment, usually at their facility, with their captive physician; you have no choice of physician or hospital. And a major study in the 1960s showed that there was no real reduction of cost for this trade-off. Another study did show that you were far less likely to have risky surgery in an HMO; after all, HMOs save money by avoiding surgery. In the usual HMO situation the physician makes money only by avoiding surgery. Thus, the incidence of gall bladder removal is 1.3 times as great in Blue Cross/Blue Shield-covered persons as in an HMO. But less risky surgery may be twice as common in the Blue Cross/Blue Shield population; for instance, hysterectomy, tonsilectomy, appendectomy, etc. And in general, the frequency of back surgery, laminectomy for presumed ruptured disc, is directly related to the total number of neurosurgeons and orthopedists, not to the concentration of patients. The problem is one of judgment coupled with finances.

I certainly do not mean to suggest that physicians operate just to collect the fee. On the contrary, I believe that 85% of physicians are honest, compassionate, and competent. It does mean that 15% of physicians put your welfare below their perceived needs, or that their judgment is clouded by greed, drugs, alcohol, etc. And while there are many fantastically dedicated physicians who would like to encourage you to adopt healthy habits, the system created by the robber baron industry simply does not pay for any aspect of health. Routine checkups, annual physical exams, and screening tests are

all explicitly excluded. For many years there has been a near consensus among physicians that certain tests should be done at certain intervals. Pap smears, pelvic exams, prostate exams, mammograms, stool exams for blood, lipid profiles, and blood pressure
checks are all part of the routine; but virtually all insurance companies reject such tests as not indicated unless you are ill with a
specific disease. It is interesting that these same insurance companies insist on many of these same tests as a screen before they will
issue a life insurance policy!

There is, of course, another side to this basic question of screening. Just what is worth doing as a health protection routine? In
other words, what can be prevented? Most tests pick up disease,
not warning signs. In a healthy person who has no symptoms and
who practices good body awareness, there are few preventive
approaches other than good health habits. If you have a great family history, free of high blood pressure, cancer, diabetes, heart disease, stroke, and early death; and if you practice body awareness or
sensory biofeedback, then you should consider having blood pressure and blood lipids (fats) checked at age 30, and even perhaps
every 5 years thereafter. If you are monogamous, and have no new
symptoms, eat a good diet, exercise regularly, do not smoke, do not
drink alcohol significantly, and maintain your weight, I doubt that
any other screening test is worthwhile.

So who is using those astronomical medical services? If you are
reading this book, the chances are that you are not using them and
that you are being ripped off by the insurance industry. One of the
principles of insurance is to share the risk among many individuals with similar interests. In house insurance, in automobile insurance, in disability insurance, and in life insurance, individuals are
"rated"; that is, drivers with a higher risk of accidents are charged
more, individuals with extreme obesity pay more, individuals with
houses far away from a fire department or with inflammable roof
materials pay more, etc.

With medical insurance, you are almost always subsidizing the
excess cost of smokers (twice as much illness and much of that among
the most expensive); alcoholics and drug addicts (with expensive
detox mandated, and highly ineffective; the average unit actually has
a long-term "cure" of 10% or less); the obese (with diabetes, heart dis-

ease, high blood pressure, and stroke much more likely); the "couch potato" (with almost all illnesses being more common); and the careless (who don't obey the speed limits or use seat belts).

If you were rated with all the individuals like yourself who just avoid these top hazards, then your medical insurance should cost not more than 20% that of the top hazard people! No matter who pays for your medical insurance, ultimately it comes out of your pocket, in less salary, fewer bonuses, and less quality of life. It is likely that about 25% of Americans share the common sense habits I have enumerated above. Why should they pay for irresponsible behavior by others? This book will examine the major factors in the sham-scam which has been created, and suggest ways for you to escape the ripoff.

We shall examine, for instance, the relative changes in physician income, cost of an office visit, cost of a hospital room, inflation, and technology, as compared with the cost of a house, medical insurance, and average American income, as well as average income of executives, hospital administrators, insurance executives, etc.

I freely admit that the current national Blue Cross/Blue Shield office is not *necessarily* the problem. After all, I said Blue Cross/Blue Shield "begat" the problem. It did so in two ways: first, by making each state have an independent, supposedly non-profit company, many of which are flagrantly wasteful; and second, by initiating the principle of hospitalization to receive service. These two errors in judgment set the stage for the crisis that came 50 years later.

This book is being completed in 1993; yet many of the statistics presented are two to three years older. It takes that long to get the "final" figures. You can assume that most current statistics just reflect more of the same. The *trend* is not reversible without a revolution.

As the Clinton administration prepares to release its proposals, leaks suggest "managed competition." *We have already managed competition—and it's not good!* If you like the IRS, you'll love government intervention in medicine.

If the Third Party succeeds in its apparent goal of cutting physicians' net income by 50%, this will cut the national disease cost by only 3.8%! Why? Because 60% or more of the physician's charge is overhead, and at least half of that is the result of Third Party harassment. The physician's net is 40% or less. Thus a cut of 20% in their total bill (or half their net) would be 20% of the 19% physicians' bill.

Where are the family physicians coming from to provide care to the 37 million uninsured? We would need *double* the current number of family physicians to provide this care. Surely we don't need such patients going to specialists. And who is willing to pay to cover everyone who creates disease by smoking; drug and alcohol abuse; obesity; excess fat, salt, and sugar; and inadequate exercise?

Meanwhile, almost a third of the Blue Cross/Blue Shield companies have been accused of gross mismanagement by Medicare. West Virginia's Blue Cross/Blue Shield went bankrupt. Maryland's BC/BS is under tremendous attack for mismanagement and the lavish lifestyle of its top dogs. And Empire Blue Cross/Blue Shield has been charged with gross mismanagement as recently as March 1993. The hens are coming home to roost! And the St. Louis Blue Cross/Blue Shield, touted as the second most difficult to deal with in the U.S., recently dropped its Medicare provider status, claiming it wasn't being allowed adequate overhead. Remember that "overhead" for American Disease Insurance companies runs at least eight times that of Canada's system.

Meanwhile, participating physicians are required by contract not to open their mouths to criticize Big Brother in any way. This part of the 1993 renewal contract amendment reads as follows: "Provider agrees not to interfere in the business relationships of BCBS with its subscribers, group purchasers, or other providers by discouraging or attempting to discourage subscribers, group purchasers or other providers from initiating or maintaining their business relationship with BCBS." I seriously question whether this might not be restraint of trade under federal law.

If the causes of the crisis and the solutions I offer seem extreme, just remember that Congress promised our senior citizens comprehensive disease care in 1965. Twenty-eight years later we have a crisis which has been accelerating for 22 years. Ask any Medicare recipient how easy it has been to cope with the system. Government is not capable of offering *any* service more cost effectively than the private sector. If you follow the advice in *Third Party Rape,* you can protect yourself from the coming chaos.

—C. Norman Shealy
March 1993

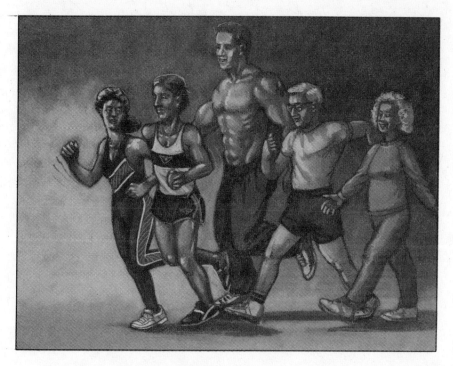

Uniting the Health-Wise

Money, again, has often been a cause of the delusion of multitudes. Sober nations have all at once become desperate gamblers and risked almost their existence upon the turn of a piece of paper.[1]

The problem is money and greed. The disease care industry, begun about the time of the Bolshevik Revolution, is rapidly turning America's "health care" into a controlled bureaucracy that will cost more and provide less. It may be too late to return to common sense and logic, for the forces manipulating the situation are powerful and interrelated. I am writing one person's interpretation of the chaos in which we live.

This book is written for a relatively small percentage of Americans, actually about the same number as elect a president! Thus, they have the potential, if they unite their efforts, to change the course of history, to reverse the trend toward mediocrity currently promoted. This book is written only for those who at least *believe* (and hopefully live) these tenets. *Health* is a result of:

- No smoking.
- No or very modest drinking of alcohol.
- No use of narcotics or marijuana.
- No prolonged use of tranquilizers.
- Maintenance of weight within 10% of ideal.
- Adequate physical exercise.
- Healthy nutrition.
- Seven to eight hours of sleep (average).
- A positive mental attitude with planned daily stress reduction.
- Belief in a higher spiritual reality.

If you fall into this category of the Health-Wise—those oriented toward health—this discussion of Third Party rape will provide you with a strategy to avoid being ripped off excessively by the Disease Insurance industry. If you are among the Disease-Wise—those oriented toward disease, the "disease-conscious," with a lifestyle that promotes disease—you may not like what I have to say. Or maybe it will push you to reconsider your lifestyle.

Third Party rape? Too strong a term, you say? Just consider these facts:

Blue Cross/Blue Shield (BC/BS), the originator of "health" insurance, has never insured nor paid for health. Originally, it offered only surgical-medical treatment for diseases requiring hospitalization. Born even prior to George Orwell's Big Brother 1984 doublespeak, BC/BS has had more influence, some positive, much negative, upon disease treatment than all other factors combined.

At the very least, the selling claims of virtually all medical insurers are misleading, dishonest, and fraudulent. At their worst, they lead to violent attacks upon the emotions and resources of victims who happen to become ill and expect their insurance companies to provide the services promised.

To my knowledge, there has never been true health insurance—a policy that insures that either you remain healthy or you will be paid benefits. Can there be any other meaning to the term? After all, disability insurance insures that you will be paid if you become disabled. Life insurance insures that your beneficiary will be paid if you lose your life.

Thus, health insurance should pay you if you lose your health. Instead, this bastard insurance called "health" (an "illegitimate" child—illegitimate because legally it virtually never provides what you expect it to pay) provides less and less while costing more and more.

And, as usual, the U.S. government participates in the Big Lie by calling disease care "health care." You never hear the term "disease care" or "illness care," but well over 99% of all expenditures covered under the rubric of National Health Care are exclusively related to the treatment of illness, treatment related to *loss* of health.

Thus, my first goal is to help you see that you have been misled—again—by the government and its co-conspirators, the insurance companies, hospitals and the legal profession—the Evil Empire.

Exaggeration, you say? As early as 1984, the President of the Greene County (Missouri) Medical Society wrote to its members, about 98% of all the physicians in Greene County, recommending that they resign as participating physicians with BC/BS of St. Louis. He specifically called it "an evil organization." Just as Ronald Reagan called the former Soviet government the Evil Empire, the Disease Insurance (DI) industry is indeed the enemy of sick people. If you are wise and lucky enough to remain healthy, while willing to bet high-rolling amounts that you may be *partially* reimbursed if you become ill, then you'll think everything is fine. Just try collecting! It may be slightly more difficult than evading repayment of a loan from the Mafia. During the past decade, the façade of the DI empire has begun to take on a complexion slightly worse than Dorian Gray as its role in the great deception grows.

Basically, the bottom line is: You cannot be certain your DI will cover anything. They reserve the right to determine whether their medically uneducated clerks will pay for any treatment, and how much. Their primary ploy has been one of delay, delay, delay, and then denial. At the same time, they insult, intimidate, and attack your physician. The most common tactic is to tell you and your physician that his or her charges are excessive and beyond the "usual and customary." Interestingly, in a recent audience of 100 different physicians' office personnel, 100% had received this lie. In other words, if every physician is receiving the same lie, it can't be true. Furthermore, these same companies refuse to tell anyone where they get their figures for "usual and customary." Two more words have lost their meaning.

And DI refuses to answer most questions concerning its operations. For instance, what percentage of claims are denied? What percentage of bills are paid partially? How much is the president of BC/BS paid? These companies have led a loud attack upon physician income but refuse to reveal the income of their top executives.

Joining in the attack upon physicians, big business leaders have whined all the way to the bank, often in years when their personal and company profits hit new record highs, that physicians and the AMA are the cause of the "Health Care Cost Crisis." Note, those words are always a lie. Physicians are not the cause; they are the scapegoat of a massive national conspiracy to cover up the bungling errors of the past half century.

The statistics will speak for themselves. The major causes of the Disease Care Cost Crisis are:

1. The doubling of unused hospital beds.
2. The doubling of medical school graduates.
3. The 50-year precedent of forcing people into hospitals to receive medical care.
4. The poor health habits of many Americans.
5. The dissolution of the American family.
6. Drug abuse: nicotine, narcotics, tranquilizers, and alcohol.
7. The collusion of hospitals with DI.
8. The failure of government and DI to provide health promotion education and incentives.
9. The blitz of the media to make new technology the Cinderella goal of everyone.

10. Special interests that restrict financial competition.
11. Government promises of complete "security" for the elderly.
12. Warehousing of the elderly.
13. Brainwashing by DI.
14. The takeover of America by the immoral legal system.

1. The Attempt to Double Hospital Beds

In 1945 Harry S. Truman said that the U.S. was spending too little on "health" care (4.5%). He wanted a nationalized Disease Industry. Failing to achieve that goal, he settled for near doubling of hospital beds and medical school admissions. Thus he helped set the stage for the crises of the latter quarter of this century.[2]

Prior to 1945, BC/BS had already set this dangerous precedent—if you want your DI to pay, you've got to be hospitalized. Between the 1920s and 1965, the era of the beginning of the Armageddon of American medicine, hospitalization was the requirement for insurance coverage of medical care. Thus the DI, in cahoots with hospitals, set the stage for the current mess. Hospitals loved it; they became the focus for disease care. From an ingrown toenail to a gastrointestinal upset, DI and hospitals provided the answer.

As early as 1969, my survey of physicians at one of the finest hospitals in this country revealed that over 60% of patients were there not because of the need for hospital care, but to obtain "insurance coverage." In those days it was relatively carte blanche. No one objected; no one cared.

Today it is widely predicted that 25% of hospitals will go bankrupt. And since most hospitals carry a census of less than 75% occupancy, if an additional 25% were closed, not one patient would suffer.

Indeed, if we cut hospitalization by 50%, we would cut total disease-care expenses more than they could be cut by abolishing all physician fees!

The biggest cause of disease expense is the hospital. Hospital charges are twice as great as any other factor. Hospitalization days per capita are greater than in any other country in the world. If America wants to contain costs, it must limit the number of hospitals, the number of hospital beds, the number of hospitalizations, the waste of hospitals and the excessive costs of hospitals. No other factor can have half the cost effectiveness as can controlling hospitals.

2. The Doubling of Medical School Graduates

The AMA wisely opposed the expansion of medical school admissions. This was instituted by government pressure when Truman and Johnson could not get national Disease Insurance. The AMA lost and so did the American public. As a result, the U.S. has more physicians per capita than any other country. The number of physicians increased 77% in just 18 years (1970 to 1988). During that same time the number of physicians per 100,000 population increased 51%. The concentration of physicians in the U.S. is considerably higher than in any other country in the world.[3,4]

Average individual physician income is dropping; it is increasing, but at a pace below that of the cost of a car, and below that of government employees or the average American family income. Quality of care will go down as physicians increasingly react to the stresses of unreasonable, capricious paperwork and decreasing living style.

For 50 years Americans have glamorized medical specialization to the point that we have far too many specialists and not nearly enough generalists.

Indeed, if Americans want a cost-effective disease treatment system, we must:

- Cut the growing glut of physicians immediately by decreasing medical school enrollment at least 25%.
- Stop immigration of foreign physicians. Over one-fifth of all physicians in this country are foreign born. In no other profession has there been such a remarkable growth in foreign representation. *We simply do not need more physicians—of any nationality.*
- Push for 75% of all physicians to become *family* physicians. Well-trained family physicians can effectively manage 95% of all medical/surgical problems. They charge less, do fewer unnecessary procedures, provide better continuity of care, hospitalize less, and, in my opinion,

offer an overall better quality of care.
• Encourage nurses to become the health promotion team. Actually, a number of "allied health professionals" could be helpful here.

3. The 50-Year Precedent of Forcing People into Hospitals to Receive Medical Care

Since the inception of BC/BS, hospitalization has been the major role of DI.[5] Most illnesses are better cared for outside hospitals. In fact, two major studies revealed that patients with heart attacks have a greater survival rate if they are sent home than if they are sent to cardiac care units. We need to reassess the role of hospitals and establish reasonable guidelines for the need for hospitalization vs. the *desire* for hospitalization. Hospitals are the most expensive and dangerous motels in the world.

At all levels of society, we need to educate everyone to avoid hospitalization unless it is essential.

Hospitals should immediately be prohibited from promoting and advertising their "free champagne" visits, their luring of patients with limousine pick-up, and probably even more than physicians, their involvement in ancillary money-making from MRI's*, home "health" (disease) care, etc. Whenever a hospital is involved, it costs more!

4. The Poor Health Habits of Many Americans

"Eighty percent of 'health' care expense is used by 20% of the public," according to Stan Talcott. Although that may be a slight exaggeration, the facts are clear:[6]

• Smokers have lifetime medical expenses that are at least 1.86 times those of non-smokers. Furthermore, they contribute significantly to disease in others: spouses, children, co-workers, and friends. Thus, smokers should be required to pay at least twice as much as non-smokers for

---

*MRI is a procedure, Magnetic Resonance Imaging, which gives an excellent detailed image of the brain or spine. The typical cost for an MRI is $1,000 or more (1993).

Disease Insurance.

- Alcoholics also use a disproportionate amount of medical/surgical care and are the leading cause of death through alcohol-caused accidents in children under 15 years of age. As William Lee Wilbanks has emphasized in his revealing article, "The New Obscenity," alcoholism ultimately represents a poor excuse for lack of will power.[7] The greatest single cost of disease care for many companies is alcohol and drug treatment. The really sad aspect of this frequent waste of money is the tremendous failure rate of these expensive programs, usually done inpatient. Up to 75% or more of alcoholics and drug addicts have failed to benefit from such treatment. Indeed, if the failure rate for any other treatment were nearly as great, it would probably be banned! Alcoholics and drug addicts should be required to pay at least half of their treatment costs.
- Obesity is another of the great American illnesses. At least 30% of Americans are fat. Individuals more than 15% over their ideal weight should pay at least 30% more for Disease Insurance.
- Excess fat, salt, and sugar are national addictions. While it may be difficult to rate the "insured" risk on this score, be aware that all three contribute to overall illness.
- Inadequate physical exercise is another American pastime that contributes to obesity, diabetes, high blood pressure, heart disease, cancer, and depression. In fact, adequate physical exercise may be the greatest health insurance anyone can have!

A *minimum* of 80% of all major illness is the result of smoking, drinking, or drug addiction, obesity, and failure to exercise. If Americans would cut out these unhealthy habits, we could cut the number of hospital beds by 80%, cut the number of physicians 75 to 80%, and cut our national disease expense by about 75%.

Who is responsible for the cost of disease? Those with crummy health habits, using hospitals to treat disease, much of which is preventable.

5. The Dissolution of the American Family

In the past quarter century, one of the greatest social changes of all times has taken place. Today well over half of all children are raised with only one of their natural parents. The roots of psychological stress begin in childhood, perhaps prior to birth. The major poor health habits enumerated earlier are considerably greater in those "families" where there are not two concerned, intelligent, loving parents. If we are to cut the disease expense model, America must find a way to restore social security through stable family units. Ultimately, the disease cost will accelerate until this devastating trend of "no family" is reversed.

6. Drug Abuse—Nicotine, Narcotics, Tranquilizers, and Alcohol

Drug abuse is closely related to family dissolution, and virtually always due at least to family stress, nicotine, alcohol, and narcotic abuse. It can ultimately be controlled only through extensive education and a general public attitude that encourages and enhances health. At the same time, tranquilizer abuse must be stopped. There should be federal and state restrictions that preclude long-term prescription of benzodiazapines. These dangerous drugs convert anxiety to depression and undoubtedly stand next to alcohol, nicotine, and narcotics in creating disease.[8] Indeed, if we taxed cigarettes $5.00 per pack, we could probably do more to cut disease costs than cold be accomplished by cutting *all* physician costs. If we legalized and heavily taxed marijuana and cocaine, we could cut disease costs and begin to win the drug war.

7. The Collusion of Hospitals with DI

Hospitals *began* Disease Insurance.[9] BC/BS quickly took over and pushed their brand of communism, so much so that the federal government was taken over in the 1965 Medicare coup, which gave DI the ultimate power. Medicare was tied into the hospital as tightly as had been most other disease care. Hospitals quickly saw the pot of gold, and a new breed of bureaucrat took over—hospital administrators. Patient advocacy was lost in the shuffle, and with it much of the compassionate care identified with healing. Working in cooperation with DI, hospitals expanded their roles tremendously and became the brokers who threw physicians to the wolves to preserve their power.

Prior to Medicare there was relatively little competition to BC/BS. But the robber barons saw the great opportunity and DI expanded rapidly and pervasively.

Prior to 1965, there were few proprietary hospitals; the profit potential of Medicare led to tremendous growth of the money-hungry mongers who have done nothing except give all hospital administrators greed-satisfying techniques for bilking everyone. "Non-profit" hospitals now have greater profit margins than General Motors!

8. The Failure of Government and DI to Provide Health Promotion Education and Incentives

Despite modest lip service to health promotion, the real meaning comes through frequently. Even our prestigious *New England Journal of Medicine* once let slip an article on "Preventive Health." Thank you very much, but Americans seem to be doing quite well preventing health without any inside help! What we need is preventive disease and preventive medicine.

Or take the attitude of one medical school professor, attacking holistic medicine, when he said we're too busy taking care of sickness to be bothered with trying to prevent it. Those in the holistic movement were also criticized for speaking too well! Apparently, anyone who speaks clearly is a threat to the doublespeak DI and "traditionalists." It's a sad state of affairs when physicians are criticized for doing their primary job as teachers.

Indeed, the major role of physicians in contributing to the disease cost crisis is in abdicating their responsibility for insisting upon health promotion as the foundation for health insurance! Since government and DI took over the responsibility for disease care, they have also been negligent in failing to make health promotion a top priority.

9. The Media Blitz to Make New Technology Everyone's Cinderella Goal

The role of the media may be more difficult to prove. The greatest problem has been premature announcements of new technological wonders, whetting the appetite of Americans for the latest wonder drug or procedure two to ten years before it becomes reality. Heart, lung, and liver transplants are typical examples of highly experimental procedures that offer unrealistic hope at remarkable expense. Secondly, the media has glamorized remarkably risky procedures that have low success rates and high complication rates. Most of these procedures are not ones I would consider. Although new technology is sometimes considered a relatively small part of the total cost of disease care, cutting that 10% would be a great boon. Saving a billion here and a billion there soon adds up!

Should *you* pay for highly experimental new technology such as heart, liver, and/or lung transplants?

Would you go through the torture of immune suppression by chemotherapy for the rest of your life in order to have a chance of surviving a few months or years? Where does quality of life end and length begin? If someone wants an experimental procedure such as a liver transplant, who should pay? Why should your Disease Insurance rates go up to subsidize such practices?

Even more critical, where do you draw the line in new surgical approaches?

Coronary artery bypass surgery, easily the greatest single contributor to the crisis in disease cost, has been a highly controversial and abused procedure. There is no common surgical procedure that would survive with a 12% success rate. If a surgeon removed a normal appendix 80+% of the time, he or she would be banned. Death rates vary from less than 1% to 25%, depending on hospital and surgeon. And at least two major scientific studies concluded that less than 12% of such recipients were good candidates for this procedure.[10] I've threatened to have the words "Do Not Open" tattooed on my chest.

Furthermore, Dr. Dean Ornish of the University of California, San Francisco, has demonstrated reversal of coronary atherosclerosis with adoption of good health habits—much more cost effective!

Here again, if you are one of the exceptional, wise people for whom I am writing, you are subsidizing the poor health habits of others when you contribute your unfair share to such procedures.

10. Special Interests That Restrict Financial Competition

Here is an area where physicians have been accessories in the conspiracy to avoid health promotion. By joining with all licensed groups to prevent outsiders, nonphysicians, from delivering health care, physicians have been part of the disease-cost crisis. While neglecting health promotion themselves, they, along with most other licensed professions, have lobbied to prevent anyone else from entering the empty stadium. In other words, physicians have cooperated with DI in restricting health promotion by nurses and other health providers.

Despite the fact that licensure in general is a restraint of trade, and not a guarantee of quality, government and the public have accepted the flawed concept of licensure with broad restrictions.[11] Indeed, the U.S. has by far the most restrictive disease treatment system in the world. England and Europe are much wiser in allowing and encouraging homeopathy, spiritual healing, and many alternatives.

Actually, in today's world, what is the role of the physician? I believe my greatest teacher, Dr. Eugene A. Stead, Jr., Chairman of the Department of Medicine at Duke University, summed it up best. The physician should stand at the door and serve as a triage officer. He or she should be certain that a patient does not *need* drugs or surgery to save a life. When there is no serious medical/surgical problem, the patient should be allowed to choose from the wares offered by all individuals who can prove a good standard of safety.

The question of efficacy should be left to the recipient. As Dr. Herb Benson emphasized in a landmark article, "Angina Pectoris and the Placebo Effect," no treatment for angina has been better scientifically than placebo.[12]

And many "placebo" approaches were 85% or more effective for many years, when the physician involved was an enthusiast.

As Sir William Osler, the father of American medicine, emphasized, far more important than what the physician does is the belief of both patient and physician in what the physician does.[13]

In general, since medicine, government, and DI have abandoned health promotion, we need a new class of quality health promoters. With the closure of 50% of hospitals, great numbers of nurses could be quickly mobilized to provide a powerful health-promotion program.

11. Government Promises of Complete "Security" for the Elderly

Medicare was a lie from the beginning, as was Social Security. The two must either be radically revised or they will bankrupt the country.

First, Medicare failed to use common sense in minimizing hospitalization from its beginning. Second, it promised too much to too many. Third, its rules change monthly, if not more frequently, overwhelming physicians with their complexity, threatening and intimidating physicians, capriciously withholding critical information, applying rules retrospectively, and working hand-in-hand with DI to encourage the greatest administrative overhead of any disease-care system in the world.

Does anyone know of any government program that runs more cost effectively than free enterprise (the latter hardly known for its penny pinching)? The Grace Commission, appointed by the president to investigate government waste and then ignored, has emphasized the phenomenal waste of government. Indeed, if government were run efficiently, not only would the deficit be abolished, but a big hunk of disease care could be subsidized. In fact, the government has provided the example of waste that pervades American industry, including the hospital system.

12. Warehousing of the Elderly

The entire concept of segregating the elderly in nursing and retirement homes is a 20th-century abreaction, experienced to such a degree in no other country. The elderly are made more isolated, debilitated, and confused by being segregated from the stimulation of multiple generations. Sadly, many elderly persons move to retirement communities at great expense and trouble, realizing too late the emptiness of an age-segregated environment. Frankly, if anyone tried to put me in such a facility while I was conscious, I'd at least haunt them.

13. Brainwashing by DI

The culpability of DI is one of pervasive misinformation and disinformation. They promise the moon and provide hell to many people. As long as you pay their exorbitant fees and don't use the system, they are as upbeat as an auctioneer. Put in a claim and you become as welcome as the FBI's most wanted criminal. Horror stories abound. A few are in this book. As Stan Talcott, J.D., said at the 1991 annual meeting of the American Academy of Pain Management, "You can have anything you want" is the selling motto of the DI.

The performance motto is "But we won't pay for it."

14. The ILL-egalization of America

The ILL-egalization of America is so rampant that it deserves an entire chapter.

Who is the Third Party?

Disease insurance, government, lawyers, and hospitals.

Why rape?

Offering the public "health care," the Third Party provides some disease care, at great expense, and even greater psychological attack.

A Conspiracy?

A major question to be considered is whether there is a *conspiracy* of the Third Party. The evidence for a conspiracy among Blue Cross/Blue Shield and hospitals is striking. After all, hospitals started the concept of Blue Cross/Blue Shield; for 60 years Blue Cross/Blue Shield policies pushed people into hospitals to be "covered." Hospitals have been much more exempt from cost regulations than physicians, and are paid by insurance companies much sooner than are physicians.

Whether they gather secretly to conspire, the entire Third Party is guilty of *blaming* physicians for the high cost of medical care. At the same time, the Third Party implies or states that the cost of disease care is the most inflationary item in the U.S. economy. *What lies!* Over the past decade inflation has been led by:

• Legal services

- Government
- Insurance
- Medical insurance/hospitals
- Overall disease care

Why is the Third Party not alarmed by the top four inflationary issues?

Indeed, although physician charges have gone up, physician overhead to cope with Third Party nonsense has grown so significantly that *net* physician income has gone down.

At the same time, no one is addressing the real causes of escalating disease costs—lifestyle and disease habits. Ultimately, disease costs are the result of:

- Smoking
- Alcohol and drug abuse
- Obesity
- Excess fat, salt, and sugar
- Inadequate physical exercise

Until these disease habits are stopped—medical treatment for their consequences rationed and charged to the offenders—there can be no decrease in the cost of disease care.

As of April 5, 1993, the AMA has officially stated that "the greatest savings are going to occur in health care reform: ... to avoid the necessity for visiting physicians and hospitals."[14]

Notes—Chapter 1

1. MacKay, Charles, *Extraordinary Popular Delusions and the Madness of Crowds* (New York: Bonanza Books, 1980). (original pub. London: Richard Bentley, 1841)

2. Starr, Paul, *The Social Transformation of American Medicine* (New York: Basic Books, 1982).

3. Ibid.

4. *Health United States 1990* (Hyattsville, MD: U.S. Department of Health & Human Services, 1991).

5. Starr, *Social Transformation of American Medicine.*

6. *Healthy People: The Surgeon General's Report on Health Promotion and Disease Prevention* (Washington, DC: United States Department of Health, Education, and Welfare, 1979).

7. Wilbanks, William L., "The New Obscenity," *Vital Speeches of the Day* (August 16, 1988): 658–664.

8. Ibid.

9. Starr, *Social Transformation of American Medicine.*

10. Robin, Eugene D., *Matters of Life and Death: Risks Versus Benefits of Medical Care* (New York: W.H. Freeman, 1984).

11. Gross, Stanley, *Of Foxes and Henhouses* (Westpoint, CT: Quorum Books, 1984).

12. Benson, Herb, "Angina Pectoris and the Placebo Effect." *New England Journal of Medicine* 300:25 (June 21, 1979): 1424–1429.

13. Osler, Sir William, *Aequanimitas*, 3rd edition (Philadelphia: The Blakiston Company, 1943).

14. *AMA News* (April 3, 1993): 16.

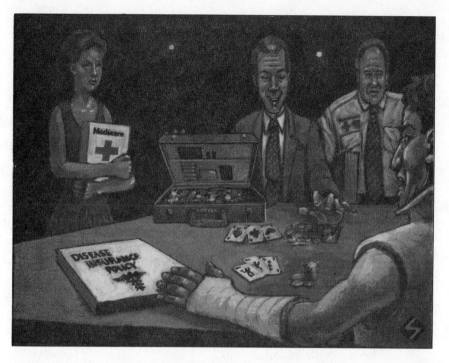

2

The ILL-egalization
of America

*You delight in laying down laws, but you delight more in
breaking them. Like children playing by the ocean who
build sand towers with constancy and then destroy them
with laughter.*[1]

The statistics about disease care are staggering. At the same
time they are grossly distorted by the legal-insurance-government
bureaucracy that has chosen to use physicians as the scapegoat,
with the complicity of the hospitals, which have thus multiplied
their power. Just look at the figures:

From 1981 to 1988:

The U.S. population increased about 7%.

Hospital costs increased 800%.

The number of physicians increased 51% per 100,000 population.

The number of nurses increased 65% per 100,000 population.

The total number of those employed in disease care increased 214%.

Just between 1980 and 1987:

Average income per capita increased 56%.

CPI increased 46%.

Physician income increased 39%.

(Thus, net physician income fell compared to the rest of society.)

New house costs increased 30%.

Physician billings increased 84% (but all the increase and more went to paperwork and insurance).

Total personal income increased 80%.

The gross national product increased 79%.

All government revenue increased 70%.

All government spending increased 86%.

The government debt increased 157%.

Total hospital admissions decreased 13%.

Hospital costs per inpatient days increased 230%.

The number of hospital employees per 100 patients increased 134%.

Average hospital room rates increased 120%.

Total medical expenses increased 118%.

Medical insurance premiums increased 118%.

Medical malpractice costs increased approximately 348%.

The number of malpractice claims increased approximately 200%.

Total legal services increased 348%.[2]

Note that malpractice insurance and legal services led the pack. Note also that physicians were second lowest after new homes and much lower in relation to inflation than anything legal or hospital-related. Average physician income is below that of members of Congress; it is less than 25% of the average major league baseball player.

Is quality medical care of value to you? If so, you are not likely to receive it from institutionalized medicine. Furthermore, remember that in the government medical system, the Veterans Administration hospitals, costs are between 2.5 (surgical patients) and 3.0 (medical patients) times those of a private hospital. In V.A. hospitals, where I rotated in my Massachusetts General Hospital neurosurgical residency, *elective* surgery could not begin after 12:00 noon; "normal" hospitals function a full working day. The waste of government medicine may bring down physician income. It will certainly increase costs and decrease quality.

The bottom line is that the major reason for increased costs of disease care is the ILL-egalization of America. The legal takeover of our society is unprecedented and essentially represents a peaceful coup. Note that the 348% increase in legal expenses in just seven years is not just in medicine; it pervades all levels of society.

The ILL-egalization is so pervasive that we have more lawyers and more lawsuits than any other country in the world. In fact, we have more lawyers than the entire rest of the world combined.

This "legal" infiltration becomes the ultimate stun-gun of the Third Party mafia and, of course, of the government, burdened with a surplus of attorneys. It stifles all levels of society.

The increases in physician costs are virtually all the result of the increased legal-driven paper deluge that is now bureaucratizing American medicine. There are literally many thousands of regulations coming out of Washington. No physician could possibly keep up with the mandates.

In a given year, I receive over 100 "new" regulations from Medicare alone, all arriving with bold print threats of legal actions if I fail to comply, with fines of $10,000 and up for failure to provide some minor bit of information such as a CPT* code number acceptable to the person who reviews claims submitted. The intimidation is unbelievable.

Escalating malpractice insurance and the paper bureaucracy are the resultant major contributors to increased physician costs.

Deciphering the marked increase in hospital costs (that significantly exceed those of physicians), is more difficult. Hospital costs have increased because of:

- increased personnel;
- increased technology;
- increased attempts to avoid legal actions by excessive testing;
- increased documentation, or the paper mountain syndrome.

Obviously, other factors are part of the whole mess, fueled significantly by malpractice claims. On the other hand, just as hospitals have "cooperated" with the Third Party robber barons, they have also cooperated with the legal system to take advantage of physicians. To limit their liability, hospitals frequently engage in a form of plea bargaining, offering to pay a limited liability out-of-court and throwing physicians to the legal wolves for the unlimited claims.

The Third Party DI has also cooperated fully with the legal profession, often settling ridiculous claims to avoid going to trial. Three personal experiences with the Third Party legal complex may help explain the complex issues involved.

Case 1

In 1972 I was sued on the *res ipsa loquintur* doctrine—"the thing speaks for itself." The basis for the suit was the occurrence of a hip fracture in an approximately 60-year-old woman admitted to the

---

*Current Procedural Terminology—a systematic listing and coding of procedures and services performed by physicians for billing purposes.

hospital for management of facial pain. She had been totally bedridden for eight years and had severe osteoporosis. Spontaneous fractures are common in such patients, with osteoporotic bones so weak that hips can fracture from normal movement.

The case went through two and one-half days of court trial with no medical witnesses against me. The judge then threw the case out as having no foundation. The patient and her attorneys appealed to the state appellate court, where the case was again dismissed. (Note that this case took place before the major Ill-egalization of society, which gained steam in the mid 1970s. But this type of frivolous suit is rampant today.)

Case 2

In 1979, the aunt and husband of a patient initiated a lawsuit, initially for malpractice. In this situation, I had performed, in 1971, an hypophysectomy (removal of pituitary gland) on a young woman with severe diabetic retinopathy. She was sent to me by the chief of ophthalmology of a major university, specifically for the hypophysectomy. The patient did well initially after the surgery and died in 1976 from an infected foot, a complication of her diabetes.

Three years later, the aunt and husband instituted this remarkable suit initially on the basis of malpractice. The malpractice aspect was dismissed and they then sued on the basis of fraud. Their claim was that I had done the operation as part of an attempt to produce a super-race in which people with diabetes would not be allowed to reproduce! I'd have wiped out my own family if that were true, as I have many diabetic relatives on both sides. This case then dragged on—and on—and on. Depositions were taken and repeated. Postponements took place over and over.

Asking for a million dollars, the aunt and husband and their attorney called me every imaginable criminal name. Finally, 17 years after the original operation, I flew 700 miles for the court case and spent long hours preparing with my attorneys. The morning of the trial I arrived at the court house to be told the case had been settled out of court—for the attorney fees of the aunt and husband! The aunt had the gall to come up smiling and ask, "How are your beautiful wife and dear children?" The only ones who benefited from this sham were the attorneys.

Case 3

In the summer of 1982, two brothers slammed into a tree a half-mile from our Wisconsin farm home. These brothers had had many scrapes with the law, and the brother seen driving by a neighbor one minute before the crash had had his driver's license suspended for repeated offenses. They claimed the other brother was driving and sued us because they said our dogs had run into the road and caused the accident.

Legally, forget the fact that one of the dogs they described had been dead for a year and a half and that another of the three dogs they incriminated was 700 miles away in Missouri with me, as I had already moved to Missouri; only one of the three dogs was even in Wisconsin.

This case dragged on several years; my wife and I had to fly back to Wisconsin for depositions. Then, just before the long delayed trial date, the case was settled out of court, in a "sweetheart deal." Our homeowner's insurance paid one-third and the non-driving brother's auto insurance paid two-thirds of his $48,000 medical expenses. My insurance company reasoned that a court trial would cost more than $25,000 in legal fees and, of course, be settled in favor of the best actors in court.

Having participated in scores of depositions and trials related to automobile accidents or workers' compensation injuries of my patients, I am convinced that the ILL-egalization system is totally unjust. You might just as well flip a coin. Delays are an inevitable, planned part of the psychological warfare of the ILL-egalization world. At least 75% of the attorneys who come to my office for depositions are ILL-prepared, know virtually nothing about the client, the circumstances of the case they are pursuing, and even less about medical aspects of injury. Furthermore, they care nothing about truth. They insert fallacious and misleading questions aimed at confusing witnesses and jury; they attempt to impeach the honesty and character of every opponent.

Obviously there are exceptions. But I personally believe that not more than 25% of attorneys are interested in justice; the other 75% are interested in obscuring the truth and winning by intimidation.

I personally believe that at least 85 to 90% of physicians are honest humanitarians who went into medicine because they care about people. I doubt there is any other profession that has as high a standard of honesty and compassion as does the medical profession. Indeed, the greatest weakness of physicians is their naiveté in believing that truth and justice will prevail. They have thus participated in the ILL-egalization of the Disease Industry by not resisting it throughout its development. It is a sin of omission, not one of commission. The commission has been the legal-insurance-government bureaucracy that has committed the U.S. to a system at least as socialized as that of Russia!

For those of you who enjoy statistics, here are a few of the important facts I learned in arriving at my conclusions, and the sources of those facts are presented. The original materials are virtual encyclopedias of facts. Remember, America has 1.2 lawyers for every physician. Overall, we have 70% of the lawyers in the world![3]

The two following tables are based on *Statistical Abstract of the U.S.* (U.S. Bureau of Census, 111th Edition. Washington, DC, 1991).

Mean Government Employees' Salary

	Male	Female
1973	$ 9,600	$ 7,000
1980	15,200	11,400
1987	24,100*	18,900

*This represents a 251% increase for males between 1973 and 1987.

Mean Family Earnings Per Week

1980	$400
1988	596 (a 49% increase)

The tables on these two pages are based on *Survey for Current Business* (Washington, DC: United States Department of Commerce, July 1990)

	Personal Income (Adjusted to 1982 Dollars) (billions)	Population (millions)
1929	$ 498.6	121.9
1965	$1,365.7	194.3
1980	$2,214.3	227.8
1990	$2,904.4	251.0

Income Per Capita

	Current Dollars	1982 Dollars
1929	$671	$4,091
1965	2,505	7,027
1980	8,421	9,722
1989	15,071	11,609
1990	15,655*	11,571

*This represents a 625% increase since 1965.

Looked at this way, the standard of living increased from 1965 to 1989, but fell in 1990.

Social Insurance

1929	$ 0.1 billion
1965	13.3 billion
1980	88.6 billion
1990	233.9 billion (increased 1759% since 1965)

Wages and Salaries
(figures in millions)

	Federal Government	State/Local Government	Health/ Disease	Legal
1948	$ 10,230	$ 8,777	$ 1,505	$ 224
1965	31,496	38,364	7,652	993
1980	90,149	169,989	71,622	9,798
1989	205,167	400,854	206,306	41,900
Increase since 1965	652%	1,045%	2,697%	4,220%

Note that 39% of the disease increase is due to hospitals.

Wages Per Full Time Employee

	Federal	State/Local	Disease	Legal	Average American
1948	2,957	2,618	1,824	2,196	2,818
1965	5,844	5,580	4,410	5,486	5,812
1980	17,628	15,129	14,728	19,440	15,761
1989	27,826	25,611	26,714	40,922	24,884

Note that in every situation the legal profession has dominated financial increases.

Deaths/100,000 population

	Both Sexes	White Male	White Female	Black Males
1950	840.5	963.1	645.0	1,106.7
1960	760.9	917.7	555.0	916.9
1980	585.8	745.3	411.1	631.1
1988	535.5	664.3	384.4	593.1

Thus, death rates decreased 36%. At least some of this has to do with the medical profession. Did any lawyer ever decrease illness?

All the tables of the next five pages are based on *Health United States 1990* (Hyattsville, MD: U.S. Department of Health & Human Services, March 1991).

Habits

	Use Cigarettes, Age 18 and Over	Use Alcohol, Age 18 and Over
1965	42.4%	NA
1971	NA	64%
1985	30.1%	65%
1987	28.8%	NA

	High Blood Pressure 20–74 Years Old	Obesity 15% Above Average
1960	37.4%	25%
1976-80	36.2%	37.7%

Number of Physician Contacts/Person

1984	5.0
1989	5.3

	Hospital Discharges per 1,000 population	Days of Care per 1,000
1964	109.1	970.9
1984	114.7	871.9
1989	92.6	646.6

Despite increased numbers of hospital beds, the discharges per 1,000 people increased only minimally after the increase in beds. Now hospitalization rates are decreasing.

Hospital Admissions
(millions)

1960	24,324
1980	38,140
1988	33,233

Operations

	for Inpatients	per 1,000 population
1980	8,505,000	78.1
1985	8,805,000	76.3
1989	8,886,000	72.8

Physicians are operating less in hospitals, but the outpatient surgical units are undoubtedly growing.

	Diagnostic Procedures	Procedures per 1,000 population
1980	3,386	31.3
1985	5,899	51.1
1989	7,202	59.3

Unfortunately, much of the doubling of diagnostic testing is related to attempts to avoid lawsuits.

Nursing Home Residents
Per 1,000 population

1963	25.4
1973	44.7
1985	46.2

By now, undoubtedly doubled because of Medicare.

Mental Health Organization Admissions
Per 100,000 Population

1969	644.2
1975	736.5
1988	820.4

The stress of life is taking its toll.

Number of Persons Employed
(thousands)

	All Disease Care	Physician Offices	Hospitals	Nursing Homes	Per cent Civilians in Disease Care
1970	4,246	477	2,690	509	5.5
1980	7,339	777	4,036	1,199	7.4
1989	9,110	1,039	4,568	1,521	7.8

Much of the increase is related to the bureaucratic paperwork and legal defensiveness of medicine.

Total Physicians
per 10,000 population

1975	15.3
1985	20.7
1987	21.4

	All Active Physicians	Total Nurses
1950	219,900	
1960	259,400	
1970	326,500	750,000
1980	457,500	1,272,900
1988	573,600	1,648,000*
1990	601,100	
2000 (proj.)	721,600**	

*This represents a 200% increase in the total number of nurses from 1970 to 1988.

**This represents a 279% increase in the number of all active physicians from 1960 to the year 2000.

Medical School Graduates

Year	Number of Graduates
1950	5,553
1960	7,081
1970	8,367
1980	15,135
1988	15,887
2000 (est)	15,774

Graduates have virtually tripled since Truman started pushing for more expenditure on Disease Care.

Hospital Beds

Year	Beds	Occupancy Rate	Average Total in Use	Average Empty
1960	735,451	75.7	556,736	178,715
1970	935,724	7.9		
1980	1,102,166	75.6		
1988	1,033,881	65.9	681,327	352,554

The number of *empty* beds has doubled since 1960 (i.e., 198%).

Hospital Beds per 1,000 Population

1940	3.2
1950	3.3
1960	3.6
1970	4.3
1980	4.5*
1988	3.9

*This represents a 141% increase from 1940 to 1980.

Employees per 100 Average Daily Patients

1960	226
1970	302
1980	394
1988	526

Much more than doubled—all to do more paperwork.

Year	GNP (billions)	Disease Expenditures (billions)	CPI	Disease Price Index	Hospital Price Index	Physician Services
1929	103.1	3.6				
1965	705.0	41.6	31.5	25.2	12.3	25.1
1980	2,731.9	249.0	82.4	74.9	68.5	76.5
1988	4,880.6	539.9	118.3	138.6	143.3	139.8*

*But most of this increase is due to paperwork.

Hospital Costs

Year	per Inpatient Day
1971	83
1980	244
1988	581

A 700% increase from 1971 to 1988.

Nursing Home

Year	Ave. Monthly Charges
1964	186
1985	1,456

A 783% increase from 1964 to 1985.

The rest of the tables in this chapter are based once again on *Statistical Abstract of the U.S.* (U.S. Bureau of Census, 111th Edition. Washington, DC, 1991).

New House Cost

Year	Cost (thousands)
1970	35.1
1975	52.3
1980	88.0
1988	113.4

A 323% increase from 1970 to 1988.

Minimum Wage

1950	$0.75
1974	2.00
1981	3.35
1991	4.25

A 567% increase from 1950 to 1991.

Total Personal Income
(billions)

1970	831.8
1980	2,258.0
1988	4,064.5

A 489% increase from 1970 to 1988.

Poverty Level
Per 4 Person Home

1970	$ 3,988
1988	12,092

An increase of 304% from 1970 to 1988.

Total Smokers
(millions)

1965	109.0
1987	162.2

This total (from table 201, page 123) is a much higher percentage of population than that usually quoted.

Government Revenue

Year	All (billions)	Federal (billions)
1980	932	565
1985	1,419	807
1987	1,678	953

These tables cover only seven years.

Government Spending

Year	All (billions)	Federal (billions)
1980	959	617
1985	1,581	1,032
1987	1,810	1,149

Government Debt

Year	All (billions)	Federal (billions)
1980	1,250	914
1987	3,073	2,354

The impact of the ILL-egalization of America is experienced at all levels. No one escapes. According to the *Ruff Times*, September 23, 1991, in 1989 more than 18 million lawsuits were filed. The annual federal caseload has almost tripled in the past 30 years, with an estimated federal cost of $300 billion. It is likely that state costs of carrying this increased load now exceed $300 billion. Thus, just the cost to all government of handling lawsuits is approximately equal to the entire national disease care system. And the cost of legal services to the federal government is well above the amount the U.S. spends on Medicare. Do you ever hear any government bureaucracy wanting to cost-contain "legal largesse"? One in six U.S. companies has laid off employees as the result of lawsuits; 25% of manufacturers have discontinued some product research; 47% of all manufacturers have withdrawn products because of soaring liability insurance costs.

Medicine has, perhaps, felt the greatest overall impact of ILL-egalization other than farming. In virtually all countries, food has been used as a major power tool of government. In general, farm products are subsidized and manipulated by the government to keep the masses relatively quiet.

Through excessive legal maneuvers, farmers have been the indentured servants of society throughout history. Milk subsidization and other government support programs totally distort and virtually nationalize farming. As a result, farmers have lost much more income in the past 20 years than any other workers.

Physicians, who ordinarily work at least one and one-half times as long (60+ hours per week) as other workers, have already experienced a drop in income and undoubtedly will lose 25% or more of income in the next decade.

At the same time, the cost of medical school has increased even more than the cost of disease care. The number of applicants to medical school is dropping, and the quality of students is suffering, with, to date, inadequate cuts in the production of physicians.

Thus, at one end we have an increasing supply of young physicians, starting with a tremendous debt. At the senior end we have an increasing number of physicians fed up with Third Party rape, dropping out of the system long before usual retirement age.

I am one of those.

Notes—Chapter 2

1. All quotations at beginnings of chapters 2–10 are from *The Prophet* by Kahlil Gibran, copyright 1923 by Kahlil Gibran and renewed 1951 by Administrators C.T.A. of Kahlil Gibran Estate and Mary G. Gibran. Reprinted by permission of Alfred A. Knopf, Inc.

2. *Statistical Abstract of the U.S.* (U.S. Bureau of Census, 111th Edition. Washington, DC, 1991).

3. Ibid.

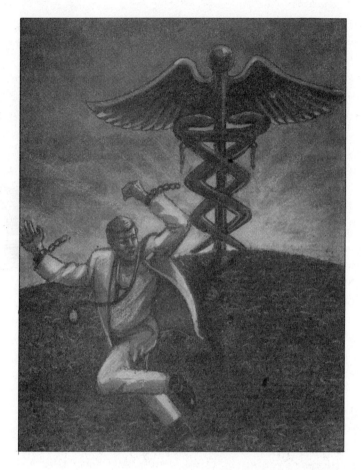

3

Free at Last

You shall be free indeed when your days are not without a care nor your nights with a want and a grief, but rather when these things girdle your life and yet you rise above them naked and unbound.

Having thought I'd practice medicine to age 80 or so, I'd like to set forth for the record my reasons for quitting more than 20 years early.

At age 16, after reading *Magnificent Obsession*, I knew I wanted to be a neurosurgeon, to explore the ultimate frontier, the brain and mind. Entering medical school at age 19, I was fascinated with neuroanatomy and spent my summers doing research in neurophysiology.

By the time I finished medical school, my goal was to be a professor of neurosurgery, teaching and doing research. But three years on the fast track toward that goal convinced me that the bureaucracy of medical schools and their remarkable conservatism would inhibit my ability to do creative research. When I phoned my long-time mentor, Dr. Talmage Peele, to tell him I was leaving academia to go to one of the ten largest clinics in the U.S., he said, "But, Junior, you're ruining your career."

My five years as Chief of Neurosciences at a respected Wisconsin clinic were very busy clinically, although I also continued the neurophysiology research begun at Western Reserve, the work that led to my introducing Dorsal Column Stimulation (DCS) and Transcutaneous Electrical Nerve Stimulation (TENS).

Then in late 1970, I became aware that 94% of the patients sent to me with chronic pain were not candidates for *any* surgical procedure, including DCS. When I remarked to a noted colleague that I thought it unusual that no physician had ever specialized in pain management, even though pain is the most common symptom in the world, he responded, "That's a great idea, but who would ruin his career doing that?!"

For the last 22 years, I have managed to devote my clinical practice to the management of chronic pain and associated problems. As far as ruining my career, I've written nine books and 200 articles and could spend virtually all my time doing lectures and workshops around the world. In fact, in 1978, I spent 180 days doing just that, although I've averaged about 90 days annually through this 22-year period.

Prior to 1971, I had always been salaried, at a medical school or clinic, so that my fees had virtually nothing to do with my income. Fortunately, I was productive—indeed, the top billing physician for about four and a half years of my time at the Wisconsin clinic. My last year there I was billing about $300,000 per year for my neurosurgical work, with a salary of about 20% that amount. It never occurred to me that anything I did had any specific dollar amount attached to it.

In fact, the crudest statement ever made to me by another doctor, about 1967, as I walked out of the operating room, was, "So, another little $500 craniotomy." This is exactly the attitude of physicians that contributes to the DI. My only concern had been removing a benign brain tumor!

When I started the country's first multidisciplinary, holistic pain and stress management clinic, like most physicians, I knew virtually nothing about the finances of private practice. Thus I was happy to take advantage of the hospital's offer to do my billing for me. The first year my personal clinic billing was about $100,000. The hospital took in about $1,000,000 from my patients. And by the end of the second year, it was obvious that the hospital made a remarkable number of errors in billing for my services. Indeed, if all hospital billings are as much in error, then approximately 50% of hospital bills are flawed, mostly through overcharges.

Interestingly, following that episode, I've had similar arrangements with two other hospitals. Their mistakes in billing were even greater. My personal experience suggests that hospital accounting is on a par with the federal defense department. In other words, hospitals waste money more or less on a par with the federal government.

The other major observation about finances was that insurance companies paid hospitals with virtually no questions or hassle. But even in the mid-1970s medical insurance companies were obnoxious dawdlers when it came to paying physicians. There appears to have been a two-tier system for a long time. Medical insurance companies pay hospitals promptly and, until very recently, without question. These same insurance companies have denied significant amounts of physician bills, despite the fact that 550,000 physicians receive less than half the total amount that goes to 7,000 hospitals. Thus an "average" hospital brings in over 800 times the amount billed by the average physician.

In the early 1980s the Medicare cost panic led to DRGs, with rapidly increasing red tape in admitting patients to hospitals; concomitant with this Medicare change, the medical insurance industry began an abusive, KGB-type approach toward physicians, denying and delaying more each year. The result is a quadrupling of needless paperwork, red tape, and soaring accounts receivable for most physicians, not to mention the stress generated by unwarranted, threatening letters from the Third Party gestapo. As early as 1989, the *New England Journal of Medicine* carried the startling article, "Health Care Rationing Through Inconvenience: The Third Party's Secret Weapon."[1] I estimate that the situation is twice as bad in 1993 as it was in 1989.

The routine medical insurance response to a claim is a letter requesting more information or copies of medical records. As many as ten similar requests delay payments months or years.

Secondly, the Third Party mafia sends an insulting letter stating that they are not paying because the doctor's charges are above the "usual and customary." Thirdly, the insurance companies deny all payment on the grounds that treatment was not indicated or was inappropriate for that diagnosis.

Fourthly, though certainly not last, Medicare sends reams of regulations, with changing guidelines at least monthly, and with dire threats to fine you thousands of dollars for minor omissions, even retroactively.

I know personally of three physicians who have been reported by an insurance company to their state medical society as practicing inappropriately. Never mind the fact that the average medical insurance employee is a high school graduate with no knowledge of the practice of medicine or even of the terminology.

Frankly, the fun and emotional rewards of helping people have been displaced for me and increasing numbers of physicians by the intimidation and near warfare with the Third Party system.

Every time I attend a hospital staff meeting, I go away depressed by the new restrictions and negativity of Medicare and insurance "regulations." I need a complex computer to tell me what is possible and how I need to document the latest requirement. Yet I'm quite sure no computer could make sense of such a tangled web.

If I were doing neurosurgery today at my 1970 volume, I'd be billing close to a million dollars a year. And undoubtedly, spending half that on insurance clerks! Fortunately, at no time in my life has money been my prime motivator. My children are grown and out of graduate school. My wife and I live modestly, not desiring most luxuries.

One day while I was taking a walk, I suddenly realized that I didn't really have to continue this nonsense. I could just quit. For the last two years I have increasingly spent time doing research and lecturing.

Thus I made the joyous decision to quit—not just retire—to quit, 22 years shy of age 80, to be free of the oppression of the Third Party system. Perhaps even more importantly, my decision leaves me free to discuss this cancerous situation publicly. Indeed, I now have time to complete a book I envisioned more than five years ago, exposing the evil nature of the Third Party companies.

So, thank you, medical insurance industry, for freeing me at last to devote my career, after 35 years, to research, writing, and lecturing. And, if I choose, I can volunteer some clinical service, knowing that I can tell any insurance company to cram it anytime I choose.

Dr. Peele was accurate: I ruined my career by opting for patient care in a society dominated by a robber baron industry.

Note—Chapter 3

1. Grumet, Gerald W, "Health Care Rationing Through Inconvenience: The Third Party's Secret Weapon" (*New England Journal of Medicine* 321:9 (August 31, 1989): 607–611.

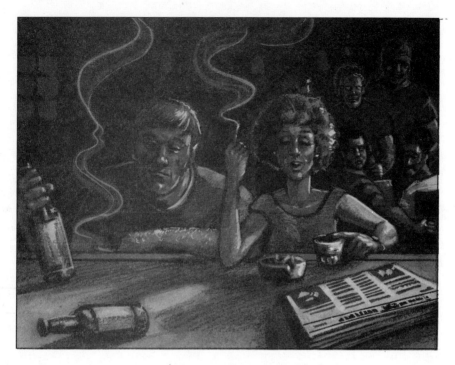

4

Who Gets Sick?
Who Should Pay?

*Much of your pain is self-chosen. It is the bitter portion
by which the physician within you heals your sick self.*

Blair Justice's terrific book *Who Gets Sick?* has covered this subject better than any other work; so well, indeed, that I made a 40-page abstract to use as a handy reference. In the last few years, a significant further body of evidence has accumulated to emphasize an essential premise: the root cause of illness is stress. From colds to cancer to venereal herpes, stress is the major determinant of health or wellness. And the reaction to stress is determined by one's individual resistance or hardiness. In subsequent chapters I

41

will discuss the roots of hardiness and the path to wellness. First, however, I wish to show that "Them that's got, gets." In other words, those who have a Disease-Wise consciousness are those who *use* the disease care system.

Smokers, who comprise only 30% of those over 17 years of age, represent roughly 46% of all patients seeking disease care. In addition, they contribute significantly to the illnesses of others from second-hand smoke. The greatest single disease cost is that associated with smoking. At least 46% of the entire disease cost of America is caused or significantly created by tobacco! Since most alcoholics also smoke, alcohol adds "only" about 5 to 10% to the total cost. Obesity adds another 20%. And the "couch potato syndrome," physical inactivity, adds at least 10 to 15%. Drug addiction contributes 5 to 10%. And at least 2% is related to teenage pregnancies.[1]

Thus, at a minimum, these avoidable illness-generating problems alone consume about 75% of all disease dollars. Add to this the fact that 80% of all accidents are due to care-less-ness and you find that you are supporting the Disease-Wise of America, through contributions to Disease Insurance and taxes.

Indeed if you are a Health-Wise person, 85% of your disease care insurance is going to cover the unwise choices of the Disease-Wise. Is this fair? Is it logical?

The question is not "Who gets sick?", but rather "Who shall pay?" If you believe in justice, then you cannot condone the current system in any way.

Several years ago Governor Lamm of Colorado was severely criticized for suggesting that individuals had a responsibility to society to avoid using resources excessively. The fact is—we have reached *the end of affluence*. We simply cannot afford to continue subsidizing disease habits.

Study after study after fact emphasizes that individuals should not be given "free" care; it discourages personal responsibility. "Over 99% of us are born healthy and made sick as a result of personal misbehavior and environmental conditions."[2]

If we do not change, "by the year 2000, the only person in the United States who can afford to get sick will be Donald Trump," as Joseph Califano says.[3]

On the other hand, the cost for delivery of health promotion averages, as of 1990, only $45.50 per year of life.[4]

Universal Disease Insurance will not cure America of its infatuation with disease. The problem is society's acceptance of tobacco, crack, alcohol, sexual indiscretion, excessive food, and inactivity. Only when society decides to stop paying for sloppy choices will the pendulum begin to change directions. "The way we live is killing us"[5] and "illing" us at the same time.

"Or is it fair for one healthy person to require virtually no cost for health through a full life while another may assume a quarter of a million, a million, or 5 million dollars of funds derived in some way from the public wealth to maintain one life?"[6]

"Individual liberty and freedom to pursue unhealthy practices and to squander one's health may be sacrificed for a societal guarantee of health care unless the society agrees that resources for health care are unlimited."[7]

"If individuals are responsible to some degree for their health and their need for health resources, why should they not also be responsible for the costs involved?"[8]

"About one-fourth of the individuals experienced more than half of all illnesses and over two-thirds of the total days of disability."[9]

Couple these concepts with the fact that *no* medical insurance company is rated safe by a major investment advisor.[10]

Disease Insurance rates are increasing 20 to 30% per year. Can you afford to subsidize the Disease-Wise? Only one-third of Americans consider the insurance industry trustworthy.[11] Disease Insurance goes to support bureaucrats who have no incentive for reducing disease costs. In no other field, except the federal government, is waste so rampant. "We will not be able to provide health [disease] care for all at some tolerable cost without controls and rationing of health care resources."[12]

The Third Party system has increasingly accepted such *experimental* disease treatments as heart-lung transplants, chemotherapy, and "unnecessary and ill advised tests," as stated by Dr. Eugene Robin, a professor of medicine and physiology at Stanford University School of Medicine since 1970.[13]

In his book, *Matters of Life and Death,* Dr. Robin states, "Chemotherapy with anti-cancer drugs prolongs the average total life span by perhaps 14 months. The treatment itself is associated with recurrent infections, fever, loss of appetite, and a series of other complications that make life miserable. During and after treatment, these patients require frequent rehospitalization. As a result, the actual prolongation of happy and productive life is considerably less than 14 months."[14]

Robin goes on to describe the problems with human heart-lung transplantation. "This largely experimental procedure is being used for patients who are terminally ill with far-advanced disease of the blood vessels of the lung. To be successful, it requires the long-term use of a drug, cyclosporin-A, which has adverse effects on the kidneys and liver." He mentions that it also causes lymphoma in a higher percentage of patients.[15]

The question of who gets sick is easily answered—the Disease-Wise. The question of who should pay will be answered only when the Health-Wise unite and refuse to pay for disease habits!

Here are some of the many statistics worthy of consideration. In the annotated bibliography, you will find much greater detail.

Total disease costs for 1988 ... $539.9 billion. Of this, 85% is "avoidable" by the Health-Wise.[16]

Smokers alone, because of their doubling of illness and excess use of high technology, burn up over $250 billion of this.

The data and tables presented in the rest of this chapter are based on *Health United States 1990* (Hyattsville, MD: U.S. Department of Health and Human Services, March 1991).

Highest Technology Costs
1987

Procedure	First 5 Years Total Cost	Number Per Year
Liver Transplants	$420,000	2,000
Bone Marrow Transplants	$462,000	2,000
Kidney Transplants	$136,000	9,000
Heart Transplants	$294,000	1,000

Current average cost per year for just these four transplants: $1.5 billion or more.

Total cost per year for teenage pregnancies—$20 billion or more.

Thirty-five per cent of all Americans in 1988 saw a psychiatrist or psychologist. Total cost—$73 billion, including hospitalization.

Medical expenses for accidents in 1988—$133.2 billion.

Nursing home care in 1988—$43.1 billion. Of this, Medicaid paid $19.3 billion, Medicare $0.8 billion, and Disease Insurance only $0.5 billion.

The 10 Most Common Causes of Death, 1987

	Rate per 100,000
Heart Disease	312.4
Cancer	159.9
Stroke	61.6
Accidents	39.0
Chronic Lung Disease	32.2
Influenza	28.4
Diabetes	15.8
Suicide	12.7
Chronic Liver Disease	10.8
Hardening of the Arteries	9.2
All Other Causes	154.3

These also are major causes of disease and most are greatly increased by smoking, alcohol, obesity, and inactivity.

Now look at some of the high-tech costs for 1989.

	Hospital Cost
Blood Clot Dissolvers	8,000
Coronary Angiography	4,000
Heart Pacemaker	7,000
Implanted Defibrillator	1,200
Spinal Bone Growth Stimulator	6,000
Cochlear Prosthesis	4,000
Penile Prosthesis	4,000
Implanted Drug Pump	1,800
MRI	850
CT Scan	700
Lithotripsy (for kidney stone)	10,000
Opening Aortic Valve	6,000

Median Physician Fees, 1989

Appendectomy	801
Gall Bladder Removal	1,029
Inguinal Hernia Repair	800
Modified Radical Mastectomy	1,489
Coronary Artery Bypass	4,834
Implanting Pacemaker	1,500
Craniotomy	3,501
Lumbar Laminectomy	2,501
Anterior Cervical Fusion	2,970
Hip Arthroplasty	3,500
Knee Arthroplasty	3,318
Hysterectomy	1,770

National Blue Cross/Blue Shield profits, 1984–1988—$3.9 billion. Of course they also had "administrative" charges of approximately $25 billion.

Some Common Operations in 1989

	Number Performed
Biopsies	1,378,000
Cesareans	953,000
Repairs of Birth Lacerations	660,000
Hysterectomies	655,000
Spinal Operations	588,000
Skin Lesion Removals	568,000
Joint Arthroplasties	556,000
Gall Bladder Removals	536,000
Removal of Ovaries and/or Tubes	490,000
Surgical Fracture Repairs	481,000
Coronary Bypass Operations	450,000

Third Party Requirements as of 1988

Precertification for Hospitalization	75%
Utilization Review	70%
Mandatory Second Surgical Opinion	60%
Case Management for Large Claims	70%
Incentives to use Ambulatory Surgery	60%

Who gets sick? The Disease-Wise, 80% of the time.
Who should pay? The Disease-Wise—80% of the total.

At this time you pay at least twice for the disease choices of others—through taxes and through being ripped off by the Disease Insurance industry. How do you stop paying double for the poor habits of others?

By refusing to participate in the Third Party lottery. Put $5,000 in a money market account, earning interest. And take a $5,000 deductible disease insurance policy. Within two to three years you will save $5,000 or more. If you are Health-Wise you can also be wealth-wise! Insist that your employer offer Disease Insurance options which save money and risks. "If it ain't broke, don't fix it." If you choose health and have no symptoms, you probably don't need medical care. The evidence is overwhelming that routine check-ups in asymptomatic people are not "cost-effective." You'll get much more health and pleasure from spending that money on R&R.

In fact, the dean of my medical school told of one of his classmates who had an "elective" biopsy of an enlarged lymph node diagnosed as Hodgkin's disease. Forty years later, having never been able to obtain life or disease insurance, the fortunate physician, having had no treatment, had never had symptoms of Hodgkin's. Not all are so fortunate. The body may be containing/healing and lose its protection *if* we intervene in a non-symptomatic illness. Why biopsy a non-symptomatic prostate, for instance? I've recently seen two dentists who had the dilemma of deciding after an "elective" positive biopsy whether they should have a prostatectomy, radiation, and castration! Personally, I'd at least wait for a little warning from the body before sticking a needle into a silent nodule in my prostate. There is no *minor* surgery. A healing lifestyle is the best medicine.

Notes—Chapter 4

1. Justice, Blair, *Who Gets Sick: Thinking & Health* (Houston, TX: Peak Press, 1987).

2. Knowles, John H. Winter, "The Responsibility of the Individual," *Daedalus.* Cambridge, MA: *Journal of American Academy of Arts and Sciences* (1977): 58.

3. "Can You Afford to Get Sick?" *Newsweek* (January 30, 1989): 44–51.

4 Davis, Karen, et. al., "Paying for Preventive Care: Moving the Debate Forward," *American Journal of Preventive Medicine* 6:4 (1990).

5. *The Impact of Healthier Lifestyles on Business & Industry* (Jefferson City: Missouri Department of Health, Office of Health Promotion, n.d.)

6. Lasagna, Louis, "Rationing Human Life," *JAMA* 249:16 (April 22/29, 1983): 2223-2225.

7. Siegler, Mark, "A Physician's Perspective on a Right to Health Care," *JAMA* 244:14 (October 3, 1990): 1591–1596.

8. Veatch, Robert M., "Voluntary Risks to Health: The Ethical Issues," *JAMA* 243:1 (January 4, 1980): 50–55.

9. Justice, *Who Gets Sick.*

10. "Special Report on the Biggest Financial Scandal of the Year ... The Insurance Crisis," *Profitable Investing* (August 1991): 14-15.

11. "The Image of the Health Insurance Industry," *Findings* (December 1990): 1-8.

12. Burnum, John F. "The Malaise in Internal Medicine," *Archives of Internal Medicine* 137 (February 1977).

13. Robin, Eugene D., *Matters of Life and Death: Risks Versus Benefits of Medical Care* (New York: W.H. Freeman & Co., 1984).

14. Ibid.

15. Ibid.

16. *Health United States 1990* (Hyattsville, MD: U.S. Department of Health and Human Services, March 1991).

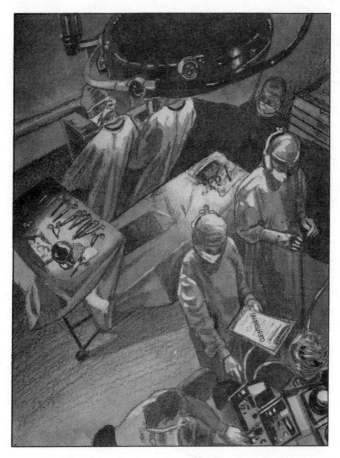

5

Insurance Principles:
· An Area of Confusion

Verily all things move within your being in constant half embrace, the desired and the dreaded, the repugnant and the cherished, the pursued and that which you would escape.

Lilly had recently been married, and this was her first pregnancy. She was only a few weeks pregnant, but she had been bleeding and cramping for days. As she entered the hospital in August, the reality of an ectopic pregnancy was all but certain. As the nurse wheeled her into surgery, Lilly yelled back to her husband, "Don't forget to call the insurance company to be sure that I am covered." (In fact, patients themselves have been back-pedaled out of the *operating room* prior to emergency surgery to talk with a DI company!)

Unrealistic? Unusual? No, but unfortunately few people have the advantage that Lilly had—she worked in a doctor's office and had been responsible for filing many insurance claims. She was aware of how many times insurance companies responded to her correspondence with, "We are sorry, but more information is necessary to verify this claim"; "This treatment was medically unnecessary"; "Your figure for reimbursement is excessive for the treatment rendered"; and so on.

Yes, Lilly was eventually covered for her treatment in terminating her pregnancy, but that is not the point. The fact is that Lilly was going through a very frightening time when her energy should have been focused on maintaining herself physically and emotionally, but instead she was concerned about whether her insurance policy would provide coverage.

Today, many more people are finding themselves in Lilly's position, but they lack knowledge about the insurance industry that may be necessary to challenge an insurer's rejection of a claim. It is often said that people buy health insurance for peace of mind and security, but what security is there in not finding out until you actually need coverage that you are not covered? I will explain the basic principles of insurance so that you will be able to understand better the cases and materials discussed herein. As one commentator said, "The difficulty with insurance is that students need to know everything at once. Similar to a circle, a clear starting point is lacking."[1]

Although it is hard to define the term "insurance," a relatively simple definition is "insurance is a technique to redistribute the economic consequences of losses from victims to the entire membership of an insured group, with each member paying the average cost of loss rather than the individual."[2] It must be remembered that risk distribution is spread among groups, thus making it clear that if you do not fit within a "group," you probably will not be covered. Although many people feel that they have a right to health care, there is no fundamental right to insurance coverage:

As a general matter, state insurance laws and regulations do not guarantee accessibility to life and health insurance. Persons who present extremely high morbidity and mortality risks are typically uninsurable; others representing lesser degrees of elevated risk may be insurable but at substandard premium rates.[3]

The effect of the "substandard premium rates" principle becomes clear when it is looked at in the context of group versus private insurance. Currently, 85% of the population is provided with group coverage through their employer,[4] which means that their rating system is based on "experience rating" rather than "community rating."[5] Community rating means that all subscribers in a region pay the same premium for coverage in a pool, thus allowing high risk individuals to get coverage through subsidies from low risk individuals. [6] Experience rating, on the other hand, allows employees to pay lower premiums because working individuals are generally healthier than unemployed persons.[7]

The effect of this experience rating is to exclude high risk individuals (such as AIDS patients, potential stroke victims, and potential heart attack victims) when, in fact, they are the persons most in need of coverage.[8] "Historically, therefore, private health insurance has never been a completely adequate or universal method of providing access to the health care system."[9]

When insurers use an experience or community rating classification scheme, they are starting from the premise "that people with like risk of loss should be charged a like premium."[10] To charge a "like premium," insurers use a concept known as "underwriting" which allows insurers to use medical histories, medical tests, and socio-demographic characteristics in deciding whom to insure.[11] This concept of "like premium" is largely lost in group insurance coverage because insurance is normally granted to all employees without individual screening or testing.[12] It is conceivable, however, that employers could exclude from coverage those persons who present a potentially higher risk for contracting certain diseases in order to preserve their historically lower premium base. And indeed, this tactic is increasingly used. In group insurance as well as private insurance, therefore, it may be important for insurers to be able to employ certain underwriting practices to exclude higher risk individuals from experience rating.

The idea of excluding persons from coverage because theoretically it will cost too much to cover them is morally repugnant to some, but the fact is that these underwriting practices have been used for years:

> In the 1860's, for example, insurance companies often refused to sell fire insurance to Jews. Ninety years later, insurers used race-based mortality and medical tables to charge blacks more than whites for life and health insurance.[13]

Although the McCarron-Ferguson Act allows the states to regulate the insurance industry,[14] underwriting practices are rarely questioned because "insurers are not required ... to submit the criteria used in underwriting to regulatory authorities."[15] In other words:

> ... so long as an insurer does not unfairly discriminate between individuals of the same class and equal life expectancy, or with essentially similar health hazards, it is generally allowed to choose the risks it will select to insure and delineate the terms and conditions upon which coverage will be offered ... a process of fair discrimination.[16]

There are indications, however, that statutes will be invalidated if they are "based solely on sex classifications ... not supported by a valid governmental interest."[17] The issue of sex classifications received recent attention due to many insurance companies denying AIDS patients access to any type of health insurance.

AIDS: Will It Have Ramifications for All of Us?
The AIDS (acquired immune deficiency syndrome) epidemic reached crisis proportion in the DI a few years ago. Although many feel the crisis has been addressed through state legislation, a basic

understanding of AIDS' impact on the insurance industry is important in comprehending the history of insurance companies and of health care practice. The DI crisis brought to a head the issue over who should bear the medical costs of caring for AIDS patients. My synopsis of this is quite broad, as figures and data are constantly being analyzed; my point is just to describe AIDS' overall impact on the DI. Although figures vary as to the actual costs involved in treating AIDS victims, an oft-stated figure is $140,000 per person.[18] The issues involved in financing AIDS treatment, however, go far beyond the economic realm. While private insurance companies have argued that insuring AIDS patients could increase the cost of insurance to all policyholders, or even destroy the insurance industry altogether,[19] AIDS patients and public interest groups have said that non-coverage will lead to further discrimination against an already unfavored group (largely, to date, male homosexuals),[20] with the possible effect of driving AIDS patients from seeking medical treatment altogether.[21]

The underwriting practices employed by insurance companies have been a major source of controversy in deciding whether AIDS patients should be allowed access to health insurance. Even though insurance companies have been battling with the gender-discrimination controversy for several years, the AIDS discrimination issue did not come to a head until the 1986 case of the *American Council of Life Insurance vs. District of Columbia.*[22] The American Council case was an action brought by life insurance companies challenging the constitutionality of the District of Columbia's 1986 Insurance Act which prohibits insurers from denying, canceling, or failing to renew insurance benefits, or altering coverage, to a person who tests positive for AIDS (a positive test result indicating only whether the person has been subjected to the HIV virus, the virus thought to cause AIDS), or who refuses to take an AIDS test.[23] The Act does not prevent, however, insurers from excluding coverage to applicants who have already developed AIDS. In addition to the restrictions imposed on insurers, the Act places a five-year moratorium (from the date of the Act; expired in 1991) "on the use of AIDS screening tests for the purpose of adjusting rates, premiums, dues, or assessments."[24]

Since the plaintiffs (life insurance companies) brought a constitutional challenge to the Act, the court had to find that the Act was

rationally related to a legitimate governmental purpose.[25] Although
the plaintiffs agreed that the Council had "a legitimate interest in regulating the insurance industry,"[26] the issue was whether the "D.C.
Council acted in an irrational and arbitrary fashion."[27] In addition to
analogizing AIDS testing to blood pressure and heart disease testing,
the plaintiffs argued that their categorization of certain individuals
was not discriminatory because they "base their decision on the risk
and not the certainty that an illness or death will occur."[28]

In upholding the Act, the court was persuaded that the testimony about the possibility of inaccurate test results, the rising costs
of care, and the existing inadequacy of access to treatment was suf-
ficient to show that there was a rational basis for the D.C. Council's
law.[29] Although the court questioned the five-year moratorium on
the grounds that the Council failed to give adequate weight to the
issue of the rising costs of AIDS treatment, the court upheld the
constitutionality of the provision on the constitutional principle
that "a belief that an Act ... may be inequitable or unwise is of
course an insufficient basis on which to conclude that it is uncon-
stitutional."[30]

The American Council decision has prompted many insurers to
challenge the Act, as well as to take a stand on AIDS coverage,
essentially on the grounds of "economic necessity."[31] The vice-
president of one insurance company justified insurers leaving the
District of Columbia on the following grounds:

> ... Let me put it to you this way. How would you
> like to run a fire insurance company where you
> could rush out and buy your policy after your house
> was on fire? What kind of premiums do you think
> we'd have to charge to people who bought insur-
> ance on that basis?[32]

The fire analogy may not be fair, however, since most health
insurance policies have provisions for pre-existing conditions, thus
allowing insurers to avoid liability by returning the premiums once
the condition is discovered.[33] Conditions excluded from reimbursement are those which began before the insurance went into effect.[34]

Even assuming a similarity between the fire example and persons discovering that they have AIDS, economic necessity alone has not been viewed favorably by the courts:

> [Courts have generally] rejected the argument that financial concerns alone justify discriminatory behavior: courts have refused to allow landlords and employers to discriminate against Blacks, Jews, women, and others, even though the prejudice of neighbors, customers, or coworkers makes a policy of nondiscrimination more costly.[35]

Likening homosexuals to blacks, however, is not necessarily proper since homosexuals have not historically been afforded the same protections as race, religion, and more recently gender;[36] history being important in determining whether a class needs protection.

> In refusing to find other classifications such as age and illegitimacy suspect, the Supreme Court has indicated that, in determining whether a class merits extraordinary protection, it will consider such factors as history of purposeful unequal treatment, relegation to a position of political powerlessness, isolation from society, stereotyped characteristics not truly indicative of abilities, the apparentness to the observer that a person falls within the class and the pervasiveness of discrimination against the class.[37]

Indeed, as late as 1986, the United States Supreme Court ruled that the fourteenth amendment clause of the Constitution does not afford homosexuals the right of privacy,[38] thus reinforcing the view that homosexuals should not receive special status.

Furthermore, the continuing battle over gender discrimination in the insurance industry indicates that there is little chance that homosexuals will be granted a mandatory right to health insurance, or even to lower premiums. Although it has been said that gender is more analogous to race than age (age not normally being included in federal statutes prohibiting discrimination),[39] gender discrimination is still justified on the basis of determining the risk to be incurred by an insurance company:

> Risk classifications have been used for years in all lines of insurance to achieve fair rating procedures. To charge men and women the same premiums for personal coverages is comparable to charging the same homeowners premium for an old frame house as for a new brick ranch. The idea is statistically unsound because each home represents a very different potential for loss.[40]

The argument for treating men and women differently has been particularly persuasive in automobile insurance because men tend to have a higher incidence of accidents.[41] In the context of health insurance, men are at an increased risk for heart attacks,[42] thus justifying higher premiums if blood pressure testing and lifestyle questioning indicate the possibility of future heart problems.[43]

In an effort to classify AIDS patients into a "pool,"[44] insurance companies began using the ELISA (Enzyme-Linked Immunoabsorbent Assay) test, which is capable of detecting the antibody generated in response to infection by the HTLV-III virus.[45] The issue of testing for certain diseases is not new. A 1914 case upheld the use of venereal disease testing for male marriage license applicants.[46] Although it was argued in that case that singling out men into a class was "unreasonable, arbitrary, or discriminatory"[47] because women were not subjected to the same tests, the court felt that since men were less "pure"[48] than women, "there (were) characteristics which in a greater degree persist(ed) through the one class than in the other," which justified the different treatment.

Since the ELISA test is not able to detect the live virus, thus not confirming whether a person will get AIDS, insurers argued the test is similar to blood pressure tests or cholesterol analysis which do not diagnose a heart attack.[49] Thus, the tests allow companies to identify individuals at high risk for developing AIDS, just as blood pressure and cholesterol testing delineate people at increased risk of developing arteriosclerosis leading to heart disease.[50]

Due to the controversy surrounding the viability of testing, insurance companies began employing other methods in attempting to deny coverage to AIDS victims. Many insurers question applicants about "swollen glands, weight loss, and night sweats— symptoms that often precede diagnosis with AIDS or ARC ..."[51] Some insurers refuse to cover persons in geographical areas known to have large homosexual or bisexual populations.[52] A person's occupation or marital status may also be taken into consideration as a basis for denying coverage.[53] Indeed, marital status is often used as a classification factor because:

> Marital status is of some importance in the underwriting of adult risks. People living in the traditional nuclear family are preferred (footnote omitted). Insurers believe that family life has a stabilizing influence and suggests a commitment to sensible values and mores (footnote omitted). Those 'living together' are thought more likely to be irresponsible ...[54]

The Vice-President of Pyramid Life in Shawnee Mission, Kansas, justified both testing and application questions, saying:

> I'll remind you that the gay community has been the victim of discrimination for generations. They have suffered and been tormented by discrimination. Do not now ask us (insurers) to discriminate against others to improve your lot. You have told us for years that you wanted to be treated like everybody else.[55]

Moreover, it has been argued that questions that could indicate a classification scheme based on homosexuality is not sexually discriminatory because "male homosexuals being at a substantially increased risk for AIDS, ... are subject to different underwriting requirements."[56] Thus, "their sexual preference, which is indicative of increased morbidity and mortality risk, merely alerts the underwriter that more investigation is warranted."[57] If the investigation shows that the applicant is not at increased risk for AIDS, coverage will be granted regardless of sexual preference; if coverage is denied or the policy is issued at increased rates, "the denial is not based upon sexual preference, but rather, upon the discovery that the applicant carries the virus or has developed symptoms of disease."[58]

It is apparent from the preceding discussion that from an economic standpoint insurance companies have a strong reason for wanting to exclude or limit AIDS patients from coverage. This raises the issue, however, of whether people with serious health problems should be looked at only in economic terms, or whether consideration should also be given to the emotional, psychological and health problems that may result from denying these people coverage. Will underwriting practices force persons with great need for treatment to avoid help, thus increasing the possibility of further transmission? Or will underwriting and testing help insurance companies gain access to information which may actually benefit AIDS patients if it can be determined that their risk and cost of treatment can be accurately predicted, thus allowing them coverage? Although insurers can charge higher premiums to smokers and deny coverage to persons who already have certain diseases,[59] it is argued that AIDS patients should be afforded different treatment "because evidence of carrying the AIDS antibody is more than just a medical fact. Such a person may never develop the disease, yet may lose his job, apartment, and friends if the result becomes known."[60] Although these concerns about discrimination are not unwarranted, there is also a controversial argument that coverage should not be provided to persons who choose to engage in such voluntary acts as homosexuality and intravenous drug use. However, if persons are allowed to smoke but suffer the consequences through higher premiums, coverage should also be provided at higher rates for persons who voluntarily partake in drug use and in socially unacceptable sexual practices. Nevertheless, perhaps the main reason for denying coverage to AIDS patients altogether is that sexually promiscuous activity and drug use carry a greater degree of social adversity than does smoking.

AIDS advocates also argue against the questioning techniques used by insurance companies because those questions "may have little reliability as indicators of the applicant's sexual preference,"[61] and furthermore:

Socially-charged insurance classifications do not become morally neutral simply because they are— or are thought to be—statistically based. Indeed, by treating blacks, women, or gay and bisexual men unfavorably, the insurance industry both reflects and reinforces social inequality. The fundamental issue in employment, housing, *and* insurance is one of access. Our society has determined that stereotypes that have polarized us should not be used to deny basic needs and opportunities, even when it is more costly in the private sector to provide these necessities on a nondiscriminatory basis. Insurance is just such a necessity, and should be treated accordingly in the context of AIDS.[62]

In addition, it is feared that excluding homosexual men from insurance pools could have implications far beyond the issue of non-coverage.

The exclusion ... can lead to employment discrimination, denial of credit or home mortgages, and an increased financial burden on government medical assistance programs. Discrimination also threatens to drive gay and bisexual men back into the closet. Although such a result may be ideologically appealing to some, its implications are medically disastrous. A climate of homophobia deters frank discussion with physicians and discourages people from seeking out AIDS prevention information that may "implicate" them as gay or bisexual. Moreover, gay or bisexual men who fear discrimination may become unwilling to risk honesty with sexual partners, and may instead feel compelled to seek the protection of sham marriages—a possibility that could increase the spread of AIDS among homosexuals.[63]

Many other arguments in favor of coverage have been raised, particularly in the area of constitutional rights, but I will not delve into these areas since some states have already enacted legislation to prevent AIDS discrimination. Due to both the lack of state legislation preventing discrimination against AIDS victims and the increasing costs of treating AIDS patients, other alternatives for coverage must be explored. As one commentator noted:

> ... if you are going to restrict people's access to health insurance on the basis of a positive antibody test, you have to provide them with a credible alternative other than Medicaid, other than impoverishing themselves, becoming unemployed and spending down to become eligible for Medicaid. That's a social issue, not an actuarial one.[64]

The problems involved in developing alternatives for AIDS patients, however, is that discrimination may occur against persons who have long been denied coverage on the basis of high blood pressure or cancer. However, as the American College of Physicians has noted, perhaps making recommendations for AIDS patients "can point the way to further steps to provide all Americans with access to care."[65]

Many people still contend that insurance companies should bear the cost of AIDS treatment because:

> First, insurers have the ability to spread more evenly the costs of AIDS ... Second, the very function of health insurance is to pay for medical care. Ironically, the insurance industry has long resisted proposals for national health insurance, insisting it is in a better position than the government to manage health care costs. It should not be allowed now to use socially harmful underwriting methods to shift onto the government a burden it deems unprofitable.[66]

An indirect way of keeping the costs within the insurance industry is through the use of insurance risk pools; approximately a dozen states have them. Although the literature on this alternative is sparse, basically the procedure followed is that if the premiums paid by insureds are inadequate to cover losses and administrative expenses, insurance companies who participate in the pools are charged for the deficit; i.e., they share in any losses that occur.[67] Individuals may generally be placed in such pools if they have received from one or more health insurers condition exclusions or premium increases in excess of the pool's premium.[68]

Some persons have also contended that the AIDS coverage problem should be "federalized" to allow Medicare coverage to all AIDS patients, or at least to those without insurance.[69] It was estimated that in 1986, 40% of AIDS patients were Medicaid recipients.[70] It is said that "federalizing" the problems would allow AIDS patients "more equitable access" to health care, and would alleviate the burden to AIDS patients and employers of having to cover AIDS treatment.[71] It is unlikely that such federalization will materialize, however, because of the current concern over the long-term survival of both the Medicaid and Medicare programs.

Another alternative is to raise rates for all policy holders within certain jurisdictions because it would force everyone to share the costs of treating AIDS patients.[72] For those of you who have wondered what relevance AIDS may have on your own insurance, this option should convince you that the AIDS crisis may significantly impact how insurance companies interpret policy language in the future. If you still are uncertain of AIDS' impact on the DI industry, contemplate the following statement by Representative Waxman:

> AIDS has shown in harsh light the cracks and flaws and holes in the American health care system. It is a crystallization of the worst problems in preventing illness and caring for the sick. AIDS has shown that your insurance system is unfair. If you lose your job—because of economics or because of illness—you lose your insurance. AIDS has shown that Medicaid is shallow and inadequate. Many middle-class Americans are learning the hard way that in most states you can qualify only if you're totally disabled and have less than $1,500 to your name. AIDS has shown that we can produce medical miracles for the rich and plain neglect for the poor. AZT (azidothy-

midine) is priced for kings and paupers. AIDS has shown that our best private hospitals are basically businesses—dumping patients without insurance. And AIDS has shown that our public hospitals are crowded, understaffed, underequipped, and bankrupt. These failures, however, are not unique to AIDS. AIDS has only shown them in bold relief.[73]

Notes—Chapter 5

1. Mehr, Robert I., *Principles of Insurance*, 6 (Richard Irwin, Inc., 1986).

2. Hammond and Shapiro, "AIDS and the Limits of Insurability," *Milbank Q.* 64 (1986): 145.

3. Hoffman and Kincaid, "AIDS: The Challenge to Life and Health Insurers Freedom of Contract," *Drake L. Rev.* 35 (1986–87): 709, 756.

4. Ibid.

5. Oppenheimer and Padgug, "AIDS: The Risks to Insurers, The Threat to Equity," *Hastings Ctr. Rep.* 16 (1986): 21.

6. Ibid.

7. Ibid.

8. Ibid.

9. Ibid.

10. Pascal, "Statutory Restrictions of Life Insurance Underwriting of AIDS Risk." *Def. Couns. J.* 54 (1988): 320.

11. See note 5 above.

12. Schatz, "Commentary—The AIDS Insurance Crisis: Underwriting or Overreaching?" *Harv. L. Rev.* 100 (1987): 1791, 1795.

13. Ibid., 1788, citing n. 43, Jerry and Mansfield. "Justifying Unisex Insurance: Another Perspective," *Am. U.L. Rev.* 34 (1985): 329, 351-52.

14. Wortham, "The Economics of Insurance Classification: The Sound of One Invisible Hand Clapping," *Ohio St. L.J.* 47 (1986): 850, citing U.S.C. 15:§§1011, 1015, 1012(b) (1982).

15. *Ohio St. L.J.* 47 (1986): 850.

16. Hoffman and Kincaid, "AIDS: The Challenge," 710.

17. Stern vs. Massachusetts Indemnity & Life Ins. Co., 365 F. Supp. 433, 440-41, citing Reed vs. Reed, 404 U.S. 71, 92 S.Ct. 251, 30 L.Ed. 2d. 225 (1971).

18. Wallace, "Hospitals Must Plan for the Increase in the Number of AIDS Patients—Experts," *Mod. Healthcare* 15 (Oct. 25, 1988): 52.

19. "AIDS is Cited as the 'Most Visible Issue,'" *Nat'l. Underwriters* 3 (Jan. 18, 1988): 17.

20. Oppenheimer and Padgug, "AIDS: The Risks," 21.

21. Ibid.

22. 645 F. Supp. 84 (D.D.C. 1986).

23. Ibid., 25, citing D.C. Act 6-170, §6. The Act, now codified in D.C. §35-223 provides:

> (a) An insurer may not deny, cancel or refuse to renew insurance coverage, or alter benefits covered or expenses reimbursable, because an individual has tested positive on any test to screen for the presence of any causative agent of AIDS, ARC, or the HTLV-III infection, including, but not limited to, a test to screen for the presence of any antibody to the HTLV-III virus, or because an individual has declined to take such a test. (b) (1) In determining whether to issue, cancel, or renew insurance coverage, an insurer may not use age, marital status, geographic area of residence, occupation, sex, sexual orientation, or any other similar factor or combination of factors for the purposes of seeking to predict whether any individual may in the future develop AIDS or ARC ...

24. 645 F. Supp., 85, citing D.C. Act 6-170 §5(b)(1).

25. Ibid., 86, citing Gray Panthers vs. Administrative Health Care Financing Admin., 566 F. Supp. 889, 892 (D.D.C. 1983)

26. Ibid.

27. Ibid.

28. Ibid., 87.

29. Ibid.

30. 645 F. Supp., 88, citing Schweiker vs. Hogan, 457 U.S. 569, 589, 102 S. Ct. 2597, 73 L. Ed. 2d 227 (1982).

31. Schatz, "The AIDS Insurance Crisis," 1791.

32. Briggs, Philip, "Should Insurance Companies Be Barred From Testing—The Basis of Insurance," L.A. Daily Times, May 29, 1987.

33. R Keeton and A. Widdis, Insurance Law §6.6(e)(4) (1988).

34. Oppenheimer and Padgug, "AIDS: The Risks," 20.

35. Schatz, "The AIDS Insurance Crisis," 1791, citing n. 59, "See, e.g., Diaz v. Pan Am. World Airways, 442 F. 2d 286 (5th Cir. 1971) (holding that

airlines may not discriminate against males in hiring flight attendants because of consumer preference for female attendants), cert. denied, 404 U.S. 950 (1971); cf. Fernandez v. Wynn Oil Co., holding discriminatory an oil company's refusal to promote a woman out of deference to company's clients, who preferred dealing with men in management positions)."

36. Jerry and Mansfield, "Justifying Unisex Insurance," 60.

37. Bailey, Hutchison, and Narber, "The Regulatory Challenge to Life Insurance Classification," *Drake L. Rev.* 25 (1976): 779, 812, citing Massachusetts Bd. of Retirement v. Murgia, 44 U.S. L.W. 5077, 5079, 5082 (June 25, 1976) (majority and dissenting opinions) ...

38. Bowers v. Hardwick, 106 S. Ct. 2841 (1986).

39. Jerry and Mansfield, "Justifying Unisex Insurance," 360. The resemblance was described as follows: "Individuals are born with a certain sex and race; absent extraordinary measures, an individual has only one race and one sex per lifetime. Although at any given moment individuals have different ages and can be categorized accordingly, age is a trait shared by all, and all individuals move equally through time."

40. "The battle that needn't be fought—The Unisex Dilemma," *J. Am. Ins.* 1 (1984): 1, 3.

41. Ibid., 3-4.

42. Appleman, *Insurance Law and Practice*, §371 (1986).

43. Metropolitan Life Ins. Co. v. Joye, 48 S.E. 2d 751, 754 (GA App. Ct. 1948), holding that the failure of an applicant to answer positively to the fact that she had previously had high blood pressure may justify an insurer in refusing to issue the policy because of the increased risk posed by her previous health problems.

44. R Keeton and A. Widdis, *Insurance Law* §1.3(b)(2). "Pool" is the name given to people classified by similar risks.

45. Kim and McMullin, "AIDS and the Insurance Industry: An Evolving Resolution of Conflicting Interests and Rights," 7 St. Louis U. Pub. L. Rev. 7 (1988): 166.

46. Peterson vs. Widule, 147 N.W. 966 (Wis. 1914).

47. Ibid., 168.

48. Ibid.

49. Ibid., citing State vs. Evans, 130 Wis. 381, 100 N.W. 241.

50. Wasilewski, "NACL National Convention—AIDS: A Big Problem for All Companies," 87 *Bests Rvw./Life & Hlth. Ins. Ed.* 87, Transamerica Occidental Life.

51. Ibid.

52. Schatz, "The AIDS Insurance Crisis," 1795.

53. Hoffman and Kincaid, "AIDS: The Challenge," 723.

54. Ibid.

55. Austin, "The Insurance Classification Controversy," *U. Pa. L. Rev.* 131, (1983): 517, 541.

56. Wasilewski, "AIDS: A Big Problem for All Companies," 132, citing Walt Whelan speaking to a representative of a gay community.

57. Ibid., 748.

58. Ibid.

59. Ibid.

60. "Insuring for AIDS," *L.A. Daily J.* 98 (Sept. 30, 1985).

61. Ibid.

62. Hoffman and Kincaid, "AIDS: The Challenge," 723.

63. Schatz, "The AIDS Insurance Crisis," 1792.

64. Levi, "Should Insurance Companies Be Barred From Testing: A Matter of Access," *L.A. Daily J.* (May 29, 1987).

65. Health and Policy Committee, American College of Physicians, "Financing the Care of Patients with the Acquired Immune Deficiency Syndrome (AIDS)," *Annals Internal Med.* 108 (1988): 470.

66. Schatz, "The AIDS Insurance Crisis," 1805.

67. Meyers, "Pooling the AIDS Risk," *Best's Rvw.* 87 (Jan. 1987): 36.

68. Ibid., 40.

69. Oppenheimer and Padgug, "AIDS: The Risks," 22.

70. Ibid., citing *Mod. Healthcare* 15 (Dec. 6, 1985): 52.

71. Ibid.

72. Hoffman and Kincaid, "AIDS: The Challenge," 765.

73. Iglehart, "Health Policy Report—Financing the Struggle Against AIDS," *New Eng. J. Med.* 317 (July 16, 1987): 182.

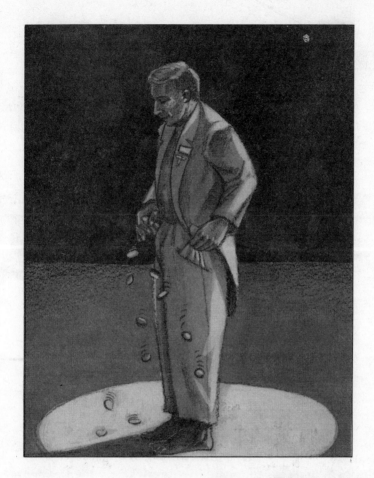

6

The Doctors:
Educated and Well-Off
—Or Are They?

And if it is a despot you would dethrone, see first that his throne erected within you is destroyed.

In today's world of rising medical costs, the doctor is no longer the sole person who determines a patient's course and method of treatment. The physician's vocabulary has changed from that of patient priority and patient attitude to one of costs, laws, insurance, and regulation. Joseph Califano said, "Medicine's high priests, the doctors, have said once too often, and with an arrogance we no longer accept, that only they should know what to prescribe, where to treat us, and how they should be paid."[1] Although cost containment mechanisms have brought to light some inherent problems in our medical care system, there has been little focus on what, if any, impact current controls are having on doctors' attitudes and their relationships with their patients.

When most of us think of what is often termed as the "medical malpractice crisis,"[2] we envision disabling and inhumane conditions which have resulted from physician incompetence or apathy. As one writer has said, however:

> Injury by itself ... does not translate into the intense hostility that a lawsuit expresses. The objective sign must be joined with the subjective state of being angry ... Without anger, an act as hostile as a lawsuit, particularly against a well-established authority figure as a physician, is impossible to contemplate. In short, the incident—the mechanical event itself—is insufficient to explain claims, and thus can only be a partial element in their prevention.[3]

Indeed, many of the resulting injuries on which patients have based their suits have been unsightly scars from surgery, unexpected outcomes from routine medical or surgical procedures, and minor inconveniences after life-saving treatment[4]—hardly what most of us would term "disabling" or "inhumane." Since the patient is the "final judge"[5] of how effective their care was, however, the inquiry should not be whether or not the patient has a valid injury on which to base a claim, but on why the patient perceived an injury in the first place.[6]

Although the literature on the topic of managing doctor-patient relationships is scarce, many commentators who have addressed the issue have focused on a patient's "disposition" to file a claim, or to view their treatment negatively.[7] One part of this predisposition is influenced by society's perception of medicine and the health care system. As medical technology increases, consumers' expectations of certainty also increase:

> To a considerable extent, while medical science has been extending its array of weapons, the general public have been fascinated onlookers. With the discovery of each "medical miracle" the press has celebrated with banner headlines. This, no doubt, has caused an unrealistic expectation by those interested onlookers of unlimited expertise and inevitable success in all that is undertaken. It has been suggested that because of unrealistic expectation, any subsequent failure brings with it unprecedented anger.[8]

Although technology has benefited many patients, it has also increased the number of risks attendant in patient care;[9] not to mention the pressure it places on physicians to stay abreast of modern medical breakthroughs.

Aside from the possibility of injury, there is also an exceptional amount of speculation involved in employing a plan of care.

> It falls to the lot of a few men to appreciate properly the effect of various modes of treatment in a particular disease. For if a patient recovers, whatever was the treatment, whether good or bad, we flatter ourselves it was the effect of our superior method in conducting the disease, but future experience will convince us that recovery, of which we so vainly boasted, was a victory of nature over the malpractice of art.[10]

Unfortunately, it is difficult for society to understand the magnitude of uncertainty involved in medical care, thus resulting in expectations far beyond that which can be reasonably achieved in the health care arena. Although the image of medical perfection increases patient trust,[11] this view also creates a stressful environment in which doctors must function.[12] In an effort to cope with the fact that medical uncertainty will result in medical unrest and the possibility of legal action, many doctors retreat into a mechanical and scientific world.

> The passion for certainty keeps costs high. It leads physicians to use whatever technology is available to obtain an elusive diagnosis, and it leads patients (who have become "consumers" under the influence of the profession and the media) to demand such diagnostic overkill. Even when physicians themselves do not see a need to perform all prescribed procedures, they may do so anyway to protect themselves against malpractice suits in which courts apply medicine's own standards of certainty. By those standards a doctor must do everything to be as certain as possible before acting.[13]

True, most of us are not imagining the fact that our doctors seem distant, cold, and unconcerned about our feelings and our true needs. But only doctors can envision what it is like to function in a world where the patient is no longer the top priority; the cost of treatment is. There is no doubt that costs of medical care have skyrocketed, but is it fair to expect doctors to be warm and understanding when they were informed at the last medical staff meeting that their privileges could be revoked because Mrs. Smith was kept in the hospital two days beyond that which Medicaid said was reasonable for an appendectomy? Forget the fact that Mrs. Smith had experienced severe cramping after surgery and was vomiting on the day the DRG (diagnostically-related group)[14] said she should be released. True, the treating physician could have requested additional payment due to Mrs. Smith's complications, but this means additional paperwork, additional headaches—and no assurance that additional reimbursement will follow.

Some physicians have told me that they spend anywhere from 15% to 40% of their time on paperwork needed to get reimbursed for their treatment expenses. Yes, many of them do have secretaries, but the demands of the insurance industry are beyond those a competent secretary can handle. In fact, increasingly insurance companies demand that physicians personally prepare and sign all responses. No doctor complained about having to keep medical records (although admittedly, some said they definitely were lacking in their diligence in preparation of medical records), but they did have problems with the fact that the paperwork they are spending so much time on is for insurance companies and government programs who are questioning the cost and the necessity of treatment rendered. Sure, the patient consented to the treatment and indeed may have considerably improved their health after receiving care, but the cost-containment era has persuaded many companies to hold payment for as long as they can keep reimbursement tied up in the mail. Some patient charts have more correspondence from insurance companies than medical records. True, some doctors lack completeness in recording techniques, but 23 letters disputing $55.00? Not to mention the fact that there was one initial letter from the insurance company saying that they would pay the $55.00 for the first visit, but that any necessary future costs would have to be approved in advance. And the 23 letters? Why, disputing the $55.00 first visit, of course.

Where does all this talk of cost-cutting and medical necessity leave a doctor? Perhaps a doctor herself said it best:

> Let me tell you what the physician now thinks as he or she considers an admission for a 72-year-old patient with severe chest pain. If I admit this patient and he must stay more days than the allotted time for the diagnosis down in the chart, who will pay for the additional days? Will the patient? Will I spend my time writing letters to justify my decision to admit and keep the patient in the hospital until I judge him to go home? Will I spend, as have my colleagues, days in court before a judge to argue the decision about whether days in the hospital will be paid for by the third-party payer or by the patient? If I do admit my patient, will I be able to prove that I have utilized my time well? And that means, will I be able to explain to a reviewing agency why a day went by when no test was performed—a test that, in

the infinite wisdom of the reviewing board, should
have been done in a timely fashion? Never mind
that the CAT scanner was inoperative that day: hospitals should be perfectly efficient. That is the only
currently acceptable standard.[15]

Note that the above statement says nothing about how a doctor should feel about his or her patient. There is no focus on
whether the patient's spouse will be able to handle the consequences of a potentially serious diagnosis. There is no concern as to
how long the patient has been experiencing these chest pains,
whether they are masking an emotional problem or a recent trau-
matic experience, or whether anything could have been done to
prevent the patient from having to make a trip to the hospital in the
first place. Who cares about the patient?

It is not that doctors have completely lost sight of the patient; it
is the fact that the patient has become lost in a stream of paperwork
and economic cost-benefit analysis. What benefit is there in knowing how the spouse is feeling about her husband's visit to the hospital when it could cost the doctor a half-hour's time to talk with
the wife? Physicians, after all, are there to treat the patient, not to
counsel the patient's spouse or family, right? That, after all, would
be putting him or her in the position of psychologist, something
they certainly are not trained to handle. But are they prepared to
handle the fact that the husband will be in the hospital again and
again because the wife's anxiety over her husband's condition has
not been fully addressed?

How do we handle the gloom and doom which not only affects
doctors professionally, but personally as well? What is it that makes
the Disease Insurance industry so insensitive?

You see, industries do not need to be torched; people and values do. I wanted to write a book entitled *Pointing Fingers: Why Societal, Not Industry, Reform is Needed*, but this book will have to do.
The concepts, ideas, and goals of many industries are excellent.
Unfortunately, the goals become convoluted in a mishmash of people wanting power and money and their perception of success.
Somewhere along the line the goals of the DI suffocated under the
pressure of egos and noncommunication. Doctors, accountants,

electricians, secretaries, and yes, even the legal profession, have succumbed to the forces. I am all too familiar with the saying, "Money is the root of all evil"—it is. A lack of communication and respect can also be equated with evil.

It is no wonder that doctors are fed up. The truth is, everyone is fed up, but no one wants to do anything. God forbid that we should forego a VCR purchase to raise our deductible to save us premiums. Or what about teaching our children that their personality and values are what count—not Guess® jeans and not Air Jordan® shoes. Frequently I question how society must feel when another ballplayer gets a record-breaking salary, but the teachers who are producing our country's future leaders are just trying to break even.

We are also the society that assumes all doctors and lawyers are rich and greedy, but we fail to recognize those who are scraping by with insurmountable student loans but still manage to provide free care or pro bono work. Some attorneys perform hundreds of hours of community service plus pro bono work, but are still hailed by some as "slimy, hardball attorneys." People do not want to take time to get to know others outside of their profession, and yet it is my opinion that until the time is taken, our values and our doctors will fall to a point of no return.

Notes—Chapter 6

1. Califano, Joseph A., *America's Health Care Revolution—Who Lives? Who Dies? Who Pays?* (1986): 5.

2. Ibid.

3. Springer & Casale, "Hospitals and the Disruptive Health Care Practitioner—Is the Inability to Work with Others Enough to Warrant Exclusion?" *Duq. L. Rev.* 24 (1985): 377, 379.

4. Ibid., 53.

5. Ibid., 55.

6. Ibid.

7. Ibid.; Felsteiner, Abel and Srant, "The Emergence and Transformation of Disputes: Naming, Blaming, and Claiming ...," *Law & Soc'y. Rev.* 15 (1980–81): 631; J. Katz, *The Silent World of Doctor and Patient* (1984): 209.

8. Bromberger, "Patient Participation in Medical Decision-Making: Are the Courts the Answer?" *U.N.S.W.L.J.* 6(1983): 3.

9. Lander, Louis, *Defective Medicine—Risk, Anger, and the Malpractice Crisis* (1978): 11.

10. McCullough, L. and Morris, J., *Implications of History and Ethics to Medicine—Veterinary and Human* (1978): 26–27, citing an Englishman's response in treating a burn patient.

11. Comment: "Healing Angry Wounds: The Roles of Apology and Mediation in Disputes Between Physicians and Patients," *Mo. J. Disp. Resol.* (1987): 111.

12. Ibid., 115.

13. Bursztajn, Harold; Robert Hamm; Richard Feinbloom; and Archie Brodsky, *Medical Choices Medical Changes—How Patients, Families and Physicians Can Cope with Uncertainty* (1981): 64.

14. In an effort to control costs, Medicare and Medicaid have set up DRGs (diagnostically-related groups) in which patients are categorized according to their illness. Based on studies, the government has set standards for more than 400 medical conditions. These standards say how long a person is allowed to be kept in the hospital for certain conditions; i.e., if a patient is kept in the hospital for a period exceeding that which the government has considered appropriate, reimbursement will only cover treatment incurred within the standard period

established for that condition.

15. Legato, "The Doctor, the Patient, and the Third-Party Payer: Three Begins to be a Crowd," *Bull. NY Acad. Med.* 62, (Dec. 1986): 956, 959–60.

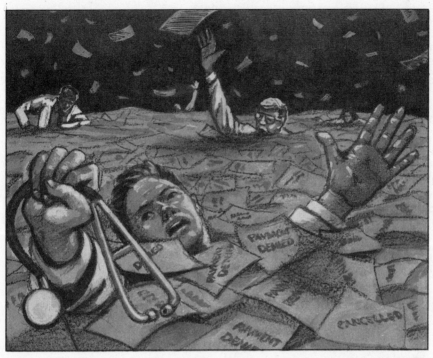

7

To Pay Or Not to Pay

For reason, ruling above, is a force confining; and passion, unattended, is a flame that burns to its own destruction.

To most physicians and many patients, it appears that insurers must flip a coin or play Russian roulette to determine when to pay a claim. Indeed, from this physician's point of view, there is neither rhyme nor reason in the process. The capricious nature of the system was perhaps best discussed in America's most prestigious medical journal, *The New England Journal of Medicine,* in August 1989, in an article by Dr. Gerald W. Grumet, "Health Care Rationing Through Inconvenience: The Third Party's Secret Weapon."[1]

The author cites the insurance carriers, "whose bungling, confusion, and delay impede the outflow of funds. For carriers, inefficiency is profitable." He states that "each visit to a physician's office is estimated to generate ten pieces of paper," in addition to the actual doctor's notes. There are many techniques that the insurance companies use to delay payment, the most important of which is repeated telephone calls and written requests for additional information and denials of payment.

There is a particular delaying tactic used by the Department of Health and Human Services in the Health Care Financing Administration (that, folks, is Medicare!) "as they attempt to thwart the efforts of hospitals to collect contested Medicare fees; some tactics sometimes hold up cases in court for as long as nine years."

One physician reported that half of his claim appeals were never even answered, and even then answering was delayed an average of 93 days.

Another major factor is the frequent changing of procedures, codes, forms, and policies. This has led to "wide spread chaos."

"Many carriers have a tendency to keep the care giver and the care recipient on tenterhooks with regard to authorization and payment for care." Interestingly, this is most common when there are behavioral, emotional, and psychiatric factors.

Dr. Grumet emphasizes that it's very difficult to get telephone authorization. When it is given, written confirmation comes slowly, and often is very different from what was stated on the phone. "American health care is now controlled haphazardly and is financed by multiple cumbersome, poorly integrated bureaucracies in desperate need of coordination, simplification, and streamlining."

Dr. Grumet talks about the Health Insurance Association of America representing 350 commercial carriers, which is only a portion of those selling Disease Insurance. That is of particular interest since it is estimated by many that by the end of this decade there will be not more than eight medical insurance carriers.

Angus MacDonald in the *Newsletter Digest*, June 22, 1989, stated, "It also seems that insurance stares at us as another cause of the increased medical costs—and that insurance makes crooks of each of us: the physician or dentist, the patient, and our hospitals.

None of them care a great deal about cost if the insurance company pays the bil7l."[2]

MacDonald stated, "A friend who was in the hospital recently was told to go home by the insurance company, not by the doctor, though he had not been out of bed and could only walk with the assistance of nurses."

MacDonald stated, "I notice, also, that insurance companies set rates for medical care and are not slow to tell the physician or dentist when he overcharges"—by the DI assertion, not by fact!

In the late 1970s about 85% of the population under age 65 had some protection against the costs of medical care, with 7% of the population covered by public insurance and 79% having some kind of private coverage.[3]

Almost all of the privately insured had "comprehensive" coverage for inpatient hospital care, with the insured expected to pay only about 5% of the hospital bill out of pocket.

In a booklet published by the Rand Corporation, the author emphasizes that outpatient coverage is less comprehensive. At that time the share of physician's charges for ambulatory care that the insured could expect to pay was 36%.[4]

Thirty percent of those individuals whose income is in the lowest quarter of income distribution lacked protection under either private or public insurance, with only 4% in the highest quarter of income uninsured. Furthermore, the poor have less generous policies. Persons who have individual plans, rather than group plans, also have less coverage for catastrophic expenses and all aspects of medical care. One of the mysteries of DI has been inadequate and excessively expensive coverage of private paying individuals. Often they offer the services of the *group* policies at twice the cost!

Although Dr. Eugene D. Robin has questioned the validity of routine Pap smears,[5] most physicians and patients "believe" they are important. Pap tests "are rarely, if ever, covered by Third Party insurance policies," according to an article in *Medical Tribune* in May 1989.[6]

Inefficiency is rampant in the Disease Insurance industry.

Commercial health insurance companies spend 14 times as much as the federal Medicare program does on administration, overhead, and marketing. They spend 11 times as much per dollar as the Canadian National Health Care System. Commercial medical insurance companies spend 33.5% on administration, marketing, or other overhead expenses for every dollar in claims paid out, whereas Medicare's administrative costs are 2.3¢ per dollar in claims paid out. In the Canadian health care system, administrative costs are 3¢ per dollar in claims paid out.[7]

Henry J. Aaron and William B. Schwartz have published a scholarly work which further compares American disease treatment with that in England. They stated, "The good news is that modern medicine can work miracles. The bad news is that it is very expensive and that many health expenditures do not seem to yield benefits worth the cost. Medical expenditures in the United States (in 1982 dollars) rose from $503 per capita in 1950 to $776 in 1965 (the last pre-Medicare, pre-Medicaid year) and to $1,365 in 1982, 10.5% of gross national product."[8]

Aaron and Schwartz began with a discussion of the attempts by the government to limit hospital expenditures, and of course they have been unsuccessful—not the authors, the government.

They emphasize that in Britain the growth of medical expenditures has been curtailed for an extended period and per capita hospital expenditures are now less than half as large as those in the United States.

Aaron and Schwartz give an excellent overview of the British National Health Service. For instance, each general practitioner has an average of 2,200 patients, and an average office visit is six minutes.

"The GP may decide to prescribe medication or send specimens to hospital laboratories for analysis, but in most cases he cannot order complicated tests or admit patients to a hospital."[9]

Most patients who need to see consultants are put on waiting lists. "Urgent cases" should theoretically be admitted to a hospital within one month, and non-urgent cases within one year. But even those standards are rarely met!

Seventy-five percent of the costs of the National Health Service comes from general government revenues and 20% comes from involuntary "contributions" by each person covered under the National Health Service.[10] Thus, it is worth emphasizing that in Britain a patient has no direct access to a specialist. The patient must first see a GP.

There is a minimal private medical system with approximately one-half of one percent of the acute care beds in the National Health Service set aside for "paid beds." There is a voluntary "insurance" which covers about one-third of private hospital expenditures and about one-quarter of the costs of private physician care, and at the present time private expenditures account for less than 5% of total expenditures on physician and inpatient care, and less than 12% of total medical care (the latter must include drugs, etc.).

In 1980 private medical insurance covered 3.6 million people in England, which is 6% of the total population, but that is an increase of almost 60% between 1977 and 1980.

According to Aaron and Schwartz, the average cost per hospital day in an American hospital in 1980 was $288, which is 3.7 times greater than in 1960 and 2 times greater than in 1970 after taking into account inflation.

In Great Britain patients with hemophilia, patients in need of megavoltage radiotherapy for cancer, and those in need of bone marrow transplantation get it at roughly the same frequency per capita as it is done in the United States.

However, the British get only one-half as many X-ray examinations per capita with only half as much film per exam. The treatment rate for chronic kidney failure in Great Britain is less than half what it is in the United States, with dialysis less than one-third that in the United States. But interestingly, kidney transplantation is at the same rate as in the United States.

Parenteral nutrition is only used about one-fourth as often in Great Britain as the United States. CT scanning is done one-sixth as often; the British system has one-fifth to one-tenth as many intensive care beds relative to population; the rate of coronary artery surgery is 10% that of the United States; hip replacement is carried out about three-fourths to four-fifths as often in Great Britain as the United States. The British spend 70% less on chemotherapy on a population corrected basis.

Aaron and Schwartz quote a leading American authority who said, "For many of the more common solid tumors there is no evidence that chemotherapy does any tangible good, regardless of the state of the disease."[11] Recall that Dr. Eugene Robin said much the same.

They even quote a British oncologist who said, "It is becoming increasingly hard to escape chemotherapy" in the United States!

In the United States in 1981, coronary bypass surgery cost from $11,000 to $25,000 per patient. In 1982, 159,000 people underwent such surgery for a total cost of between $2.5 and $3 billion, or roughly 1% of the total United States' medical expenditures.

"Statistics show that for approximately 70,000 of the 115,000 patients in the United States who underwent coronary artery surgery in 1979, the operation reduced cardiac pain but did not increase life expectancy. Of the remaining 44,000 patients, perhaps 5,000 who would have died without surgery were alive after five years."[12]

We do approximately nine times as many coronary bypasses in the United States as are done in England; and, interestingly, more people die from coronary heart disease in the United States than in the United Kingdom.

In 1978, total medical expenses in the United States were $862.50 per capita, whereas in Great Britain they were $308.40 per capita. Total hospital expenses per capita in the United States were $327.33, and in Great Britain $173.96.[13] "The federal government has tried to hold down costs by limiting purchases of equipment and controlling the number of hospital beds. These programs have enjoyed few successes."[14] In other words, if you like the IRS, you'll love a National Disease Insurance—greater cost, greater hassle, less service!

It pays to be nasty to insurance companies when they are nasty to you. Quoting from a recent letter to me in relation to a patient: "The medical records we have received are definitely altered and do not include complete information."[15]

My reply to this company was:

Your very offensive note of July 16, 1991, has been

brought to my attention. Our records have not been altered, and for you to make a statement such as that is certainly offensive and potentially libelous. You may well have had copies made in which psychological counseling notes were not copied because in general the individual counseling sessions with a psychologist are considered to be confidential information to allow the patient to discuss freely what his/her problems are. Considering the fact that from our point of view this seems more likely a delay than a legitimate excuse on your part, we would ask that this bill be paid promptly within 30 days, or we shall report it to the insurance commissioner of the state.[16]

The interesting reply after my very strong letter was, "I apologize for the harshness of my wording in my letter of July 16, 1991. … Your bill has now been reviewed and payment will be made within the next seven days."[17] This reply was sent just eight days after my letter was sent, the fastest reply I ever got from D.I.

We have known for a long time that the medical insurance industry seems to be taking over the practice of medicine. How about this one from my least favorite of all medical insurance companies, Blue Cross/Blue Shield of St. Louis? This came in a letter marked "Personal."

"Dear Dr. Shealy: We want to do what you want to do—practice medicine. Not be aggravated by insurance claims paperwork."[18]

If any nurse, acupuncturist, or lay person made such a claim, they would be under legal attack immediately. But there was no response from the state licensing board! No one wants to challenge the robber barons, especially when the executive secretary of the state board formerly worked for Blue Cross/Blue Shield for 15 years. The tie-in between Blue Cross/Blue Shield and the administration of many medical societies needs much further investigation as a conflict of interest.

Despite the fact that there is greater Disease Insurance cost than steel in the average American car, there seems no end to the expense dilemma.

"The 1990 National Executive Poll on Health Care Costs and Benefits," which was sent to 1,500 executives, 28%, or 419, of whom returned the survey, showed, "Twenty-five cents of every dollar of net profit American corporations earn is going to pay for health benefits."[19]

Ninety-two percent of executives are concerned about rising health insurance premium costs, and 81% are going to trim so-called health programs by increasing the employee's share of premium costs. Interestingly, 40% rank physician charges and 37% rank hospital costs as having a large impact on their company's rising health care expenditures.[20]

Thirty percent favor a national health insurance (they've got to be crazy!), 45% oppose it, and 25% are neutral. Thirty percent believe it will be instituted within five years, and only 11% believe it will never happen.

The top ten work force health problems are considered to be stress, high blood pressure, cigarette smoking, back injuries/pain, overweight, alcohol abuse, high cholesterol, drug abuse, depression, and mental health problems, all largely preventable.

These facts seem particularly pathetic in view of the comments by Dr. John Knowles in 1977. "Health (i.e., disease) insurance has solidified the behavior of both producers and consumers in such a way that neither is interested in, or rewarded for, health maintenance efforts."[21]

In November 1987 U.S. News & World Report reported some interesting disease-related cost estimates per year: Strep throat culture, $900 million; chest X-ray, $850 million; other X-rays, $3.2 billion; complete blood counts, $900 million; EKGs, $1 billion; coronary angiography, $2.2 billion; cardiac stress tests, $500 million; cardiac and liver enzyme tests, $750 million; fetal ultrasound, $60 million; internal fetal monitoring, $52 million; red blood cell sedimentation rate, $1.1 billion; Pap smears, $280 million; urinalysis, $1.3 billion; pulmonary artery catheterization, $420 million; and endoscopy, $5.6 billion. About one-third of all medical costs of the, at that time, $450 billion health care bill, or $150 billion, went to so-called medical tests.[22]

In a March 1991 USA Today article, Kevin Anderson reported, "In a recent poll by Northwestern Mutual Life, 60% said they had no confidence their insurance would cover a major illness a few years from now." Anderson also mentions a study at Harvard University School of Public Health in which it is estimated that 28% of all workers will lose medical insurance coverage by 1993. In this particular article, it states insurance administration costs eat up 15% of total costs vs. 5% in Canada. On average, medical insurance cost has been increasing at about 20% per year.[23]

In two years worker-paid insurance costs have risen 70%. Interestingly, 80% of recent strikes have been over medical benefits. In 1991 it's estimated that the disease cost will be $700 billion, 8% more than 1990, 144% more than 10 years ago. Medical expenses account for 12% of our total economy vs. 9.1% in 1980. In addition to the 37 million Americans who have no coverage at all, an additional 30–50 million are believed to be lacking adequate coverage.[24]

Medicare not only led the way in creating the explosion in disease costs, it has led the way in imposing bureaucratic controls. "A program originally designed to insure that the nation's elderly would have access to high-quality medical care has been complicated and crippled, largely in misguided efforts to reduce spending. ...

"Physicians who see large numbers of Medicare patients can provide a litany of horror stories that range from unreasonable paperwork demands to removal from participation in the program for specious reasons."[24] Note "specious reasons," not fraud.

"Many of the requirements seem to have been put in place largely to complicate their lives. Many of these are unreasonable and unfair."[25]

In an editorial in *Pain Management*, David Tollison states, "I sense a mounting social and professional frustration within our membership, a frustration that is being fueled by a limited number of reimbursement sources intent upon economic sanctions against patients in pain and professionals treating pain."[26]

Tollison states, "Typically, these reports describe unexplained reimbursement delays, voluminous questions and paperwork, reimbursement categories inconsistent with pain management service delivery, administrative policies that effectively prohibit reimbursement or occasionally a company or agency policy that categorically rejects pain management and/or comprehensive treatment centers as reimbursement. These charges have been lev-

eled against identified workers' compensation insurance companies; isolated state Blue Cross and Blue Shield organizations; companies insuring state, federal, and union employees; HMOs; PPOs;
companies regulating state Medicare contracts; and proprietary
general health insurance companies."

Not only is the fight for payment of claims incessant, it is fought
with the increasing possibility that the insurance company may go
belly-up, as in fact they have without prior warning.

Profitable Investing carried an article in August 1991 which
stated, "Why your insurance may fail next ... making your policies
of life insurance, and annuities worthless. No FDIC to bail you out."
The author says, "The biggest, most devastating black hole I've seen
in years is looming in the insurance industry ... We're now seeing
the tip of the iceberg in what I predict will be the biggest financial
scandal of the next 12 months ... Incredible as it may seem, up to
20% of the 100 largest life insurers, which account for more than
four-fifths of the industry's assets, could become insolvent in the
1990's ... The reason is junk bond and junk real estate investments,
managerial incompetence, and ruthless competition."[27]

The author of the *Profitable Investing* article quotes Peter Hiam,
former Massachusetts insurance commissioner who says, "It's a
real problem. Most of the companies are not in a position to ride out
a severe or long-lasting recession."

The chief executive officer of *Life USA* stated, "There are many
insurance companies in deep, fundamental trouble. People would
be scared if they knew what was happening."

Forty insurance firms went bankrupt in 1990 and many more
are likely to go down in the next few years.

"Your claim, whether for medical bills you thought were covered, your annuity policy, your life insurance proceeds, whatever,
could go unpaid for years while you and other creditors wrangle."[28]

Of course the *Profitable Investing* article mentions Blue Cross/
Blue Shield of West Virginia that went down with $50 million in
unpaid medical bills. At least 15 other Blue Cross/Blue Shield firms
are in serious trouble.

The author feels that the Best rating industry system is too easy
on the industry. "Some companies that have had Best's highest rating later became insolvent!"

Incidentally, the author does not mention *any* insurance companies which are considered recommended for Disease Insurance.

Who is to pay when Blue Cross/Blue Shield of West Virginia goes bankrupt? The "right" to disease care is challenged again and again, even when one has paid!

In an October 1980 article in *JAMA*, Mark Siegler, Associate Professor of Medicine at the University of Chicago, states, "Individual liberty and freedom to pursue unhealthy practices and to squander one's health may be sacrificed for a societal guarantee of health care unless the society agrees that resources for health care are unlimited." He argues that we need to "resist the rhetorical excess of a claim to a right to health care."[29]

Siegler rejects the notion of a right to health care because: "(1) The language of rights provides an impoverished moral vision of what a properly constituted society ought to provide its citizens in the way of health care. (2) A right to health care is unworkably ambiguous in the absence of a restricted, normative definition of health and of health care. (3) Such a right would have a detrimental and destructive effect on the practice of medicine, particularly in limiting the freedom of both patients and physicians and in changing the physician-patient relationship from covenantal to a contractual one. (4) The right to health care would reduce substantially the liberty and freedom of all citizens, patients, and prospective patients alike."

Over and over I am reminded that this concept of "crisis" has existed for over 20 years. In an article in April 1970 in *Scientific American*, Sidney Garfield states, "Medical care in the U.S. is expensive and poorly distributed, and national health insurance will make things worse. What is needed is an innovative system in which the sick are separated from the well."[30]

Garfield argues that only the truly sick should see a physician, that the well and even the early sick should probably be seen by paramedicals for initial evaluation, testing, supervision, health education, and preventive illness approaches. But who will pay?

This question of who shall pay and whether "they" will pay recurs constantly. While we are facing unprecedented harassment by the Disease Insurance industry, the cause of much illness remains unapproached, and the corrective (preventive) approach is not paid by anyone.

In a booklet put out by the Missouri Department of Health, Office of Health Promotion, it is stated, "The way we live is literally killing us." This was in approximately 1986. They report that as of 1985 a survey by the Missouri Department of Health found that in 100 employees, 32 smoke cigarettes; 15 drink over 5 drinks in one sitting; 5 have chronic drinking problems; 3 drive while intoxicated; 18 have high blood pressure; 25 are obese; 77 do not get enough exercise; and 77 do not wear seat belts.[31]

They recommend the establishment of a Missouri Commission on Employee Health Promotion, reducing stress levels, establishing smoke-free working environments, providing a healthy work site environment, and increasing comprehensive work site health promotion programs. We are now several years later; has anything been done to implement these suggestions?

In a personal letter from Dr. Charles Maclean, he notes from a *Business Week* article that 85% of an individual's medical care expenses occur in the last two years of life, and as of 1989 37% of an average company's net profit went for medical expenses.[32]

Maclean states that Robert Blank in *Rationing Medicine* felt that 80% of illnesses can be linked to lifestyle related choices such as smoking, alcohol consumption, illicit drug use, poor diet, obesity, or sexual promiscuity.

The abuses of a diseased lifestyle translate to surmounting medical costs, gathering speed as a boulder racing downhill. The *Titanic* is not salvageable once the ship is riddled with holes and three-quarters sunk! Yet, we continue to pour money in. What will happen when the robber barons get their way and refuse to pay for any illness? Will they pay then for health promotion? And increasingly the big question is: "Who Practices Medicine Today?" "Insurance companies are running and ruining the practice of medicine today."[33]

Since early in the century, state laws have restricted the practice of medicine primarily to licensed M.D.s (allopaths) and grudgingly to D.O.s (osteopaths). (This training is the same, by the way, except that D.O.s typically learn an additional skill in osteopathic college, manipulation.) D.O.s won the major legal right to practice medicine in the mid–1960s after 70 years of harassment and suppression. In a bold attempt to wipe out osteopathy, D.O.s were allowed to "convert" overnight and become M.D.s. Fortunately, enough D.O.s preferred their role to resist the bait, so that osteopathy continues to flourish.

Chiropractors (D.C.s) were vigorously fought, sometimes jailed, and repeatedly called fraudulent until a landmark anti-trust court case in which the AMA was required to cease overt attacks upon chiropractors. Now there are over 300 hospitals which allow chiropractors some staff privileges and sometimes greater reimbursement by third parties than M.D.s and D.O.s are permitted!

Increasingly, however, it is the Third Party (Disease Insurance-government-hospital-lawyers) and their often ill-trained high school graduate clerks who control the practice of medicine far more specifically and comprehensively than physicians. At a time when increasing technology requires ever greater clinical judgment and skill, the regulations and harassment not only increase costs, they also "restrain trade"—that is, they dictate what can be done. The patient is typically the loser. Government and bureaucratic waste (administration charges of over 30%) "save" a few pennies while costing many dollars. Just as the IRS overhead is so great that the U.S. could save billions in administration by going to a simple sales tax for federal revenue that would be less tempting to cheaters as well, the government does nothing that is cost-effective. Ten-thousand-dollar toilet seats are the tip of the iceberg. The Disease Insurance industry, having virtually no external restraints, is now dominating medicine and determining who shall live.

In his excellent book, *Who Shall Live*, Victor Fuchs raised that crucial question. Citing the crisis in disease care, he stated, "We cannot all have everything that we would like to have."[34] The differences in health between the U.S. and other developed countries are not due to the "quantity or quality of medical care."[35] It is due mainly to personal behavior. "Highest quality care for all is pie in the sky."[36] "The grim fact is that no nation is wealthy enough to avoid all avoidable deaths."[37]

Physicians have lost control of disease care; they never became interested in health care. If you wish your disease care to be dictated by an untrained clerk, then stay in "the system." Neither you nor your physician(s) will determine who practices what. The robber barons are now fully in charge of the "practice" of medicine!

Notes—Chapter 7

1. Grumet, Gerald W., "Health Care Rationing Through Inconvenience: The Third Party's Secret Weapon," *New England Journal of Medicine* 321:9 (August 31, 1989): 607–611.

2. MacDonald, Angus, *Newsletter Digest* (June 22, 1989).

3. Marquis, Susan M., *Characteristics of Health Insurance Coverage: Descriptive and Methodological Findings From the Health Insurance Experiment* (Santa Monica, CA: The Rand Corp., August 1986).

4. Ibid.

5. Robin, Eugene D., *Matters of Life and Death: Risks vs. Benefits of Medical Care.* (New York:W.H. Freeman & Company, 1984).

6. "Pap Test Nonpayment Decried: Insurance Won't Pay for Screening Use," *Medical Tribune* 30:13 (Thursday, May 11, 1989): 1, 7.

7. "Private Insurers Waste Money, Says Citizen Action," *News-Leader* (Wednesday, October 10, 1990): 6B.

8. Aaron, Henry J. & Schwartz, William B., *The Painful Prescription: Rationing Hospital Care* (Washington, DC: The Brookings Institution, 1984).

9. Ibid., 15.

10. Ibid.

11. Ibid., 45.

12. Ibid., 64.

13. Ibid., 85.

14. Ibid., 134.

15. McBryan, Patricia A. (Aetna), Letter from Bridgeton, Missouri, to Shealy Institute Medical Records, Springfield, Missouri, July 16, 1991. Transcript in the hand of C. Norman Shealy, Shealy Institute, Springfield, Missouri.

16. Shealy, C. Norman, Letter from Springfield, Missouri to Patricia McBryan (Aetna), Bridgeton, Missouri, July 18, 1991. Transcript in the hand of C. Norman Shealy, Shealy Institute, Springfield, Missouri.

17. McBryan, Patricia A. (Aetna). Letter from Bridgeton, Missouri, to C. Norman Shealy, Springfield, Missouri, July 26, 1991. Transcript in the

hand of C. Norman Shealy, Shealy Institute, Springfield, Missouri.

18. Goldstein, Jerry (Blue Cross/Blue Shield of Missouri). Letter from St. Louis, Missouri, to C. Norman Shealy, Springfield, Missouri, July 23, 1991. Transcript in the hand of C. Norman Shealy, Shealy Institute, Springfield, Missouri.

19. "The 1990 National Executive Poll on Health Care Costs and Benefits." *Business and Health* (April 1990): 25–38.

20. Ibid.

21. Knowles, John H. Winter, "The Responsibility of the Individual," *Daedalus.* (Cambridge, MA: The Journal of the American Academy of Arts and Sciences, 1977.)

22. "Are We Hooked on Tests?" *U.S. News & World Report* (November 23, 1987): 60-61.

23. Anderson, Kevin, "Health Care Costs More, Serves Fewer," *USA Today* (March 11, 1991): 1B–2B.

24. Ibid.

25. "Physicians Feeling Medicare Burdens," *American Medical News* (October 12, 1990): 21.

26. Tollison, C. David, "The Insurance Blues," *Pain Management* (July/August 1989): 170–171.

27. "Special Report on the Biggest Financial Scandal of the Year ... The Insurance Crisis," *Profitable Investing* (August 1991): 14–15.

28. Ibid.

29. Siegler, Mark, "A Physician's Perspective on the Right to Health Care," *JAMA* 244:14 (October 3, 1980): 1591–1596.

30. Garfield, Sidney R., "The Delivery of Medical Care," *Scientific American* 222:4 (April 1970): 15–23.

31. *The Impact of Healthier Lifestyles on Business and Industry* (Jefferson City, MO: Missouri Department of Health, Office of Health Promotion, n.d.).

32. Maclean, Charles B. Letter from Dallas, TX to C. Norman Shealy, Springfield, MO, May 18, 1990. Transcript in the hand of C. Norman Shealy, Springfield, MO.

33. Margoles, Michael. September 6, 1991. Oral presentation at the 15th Annual Scientific Meeting of the American Academy of Neurological

and Orthopaedic Surgeons.

34. Fuchs, Victor R. *Who Shall Live?* (New York: Harper-Collins, 1983), 4.

35. Ibid., 6.

36. Ibid., 7.

37. Ibid., 17.

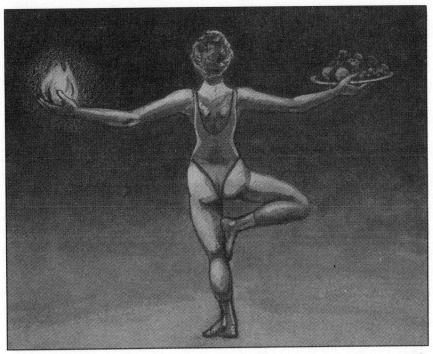

8

The Roots of Health

And since you are a breath in God's sphere, and a leaf in God's forest, you too should rest in reason and move in passion.

In chapter 4 I began to suggest a course of action for the Health-Wise: drop out of the system, take a $5,000 deductible Disease Insurance policy, and save the difference. Five years ago my wife and I did just that. The first year we saved $3,500! Interestingly, in year four our premium has *doubled*, despite no claims on the policy, and is now $1,300 per year, yet *each* year we save at least another $4,500. Our "medical" expenses have been a few elective tests of cholesterol checks and our use of vitamin-mineral supplements. We decided to choose this approach because we practice excellent health habits. Assuming that most persons reading this book are Health-Wise, or at least health-curious, let us now explore the world of health and how to achieve it.

Ninety-eight per cent of human beings born to non-drug-addicted mothers are born healthy, and the natural automatic process of homeostasis (internal balance) works, despite overwhelming odds, to keep us healthy. The expanding field of psychoneuroimmunology, the study of mental effects upon our immune system, increasingly proves that *every thought* has immediate electrical and chemical effects upon our body—and health.

Negative, stressful thoughts evoke potentially harmful, energy-sapping effects. Positive, happy thoughts strengthen and energize us at many levels. Once you realize the significance of these facts, you recognize, as one of my patients said, "I now realize that I cannot afford the luxury of depression."

The roots of our basic attitudes which regulate the degree of negativity/positivity in our minds are set in early childhood. Indeed, there is considerable evidence that the foundation begins at least as early as the moment of conception! If your parents, especially your mother, were happy and eager to conceive, you already have the greatest gift it is possible to receive. The overall joy of your mother throughout nine months of gestation will shape and mold your personality for much of your life.

Unwanted children know, even before birth, that they are relatively unloved, and they strive throughout life to feel wanted, loved, "OK" as Tom Harris said in *I'm OK, You're OK*.[1]

After birth, the first six months of life are particularly crucial. Adequate nurturing during this period is essential, and the overall nurturing received in the first six years of life is more important than all other factors in determining relative health and emotional well-being throughout life.

For most individuals in the Western world, most of the basic essentials for survival are well met—air, water, food, shelter, and clothing are obviously absolute necessities. In third world countries and among the very poor or severely socially deprived, such as drug addicts, these basic needs are inadequately met. In such cases serious injury may misshape and damage an individual irreparably.

An equally critical survival need is nurturing. Infants who are so unnurtured as to feel totally rejected may develop marasmus and waste away, much like a severe case of anorexia nervosa in teenagers. Yet in the West especially, nurturing needs are peculiarly underestimated. For example, though perceived as abandonment, infants are routinely separated from their mothers at the moment of birth. This barbaric practice may trigger in us a lifelong quest for nurturing. In fact, mothers often tell stories of their infants being taken away at birth and withheld from them for a day or so without explanation.

Other events, such as the birth of another child, maternal illnesses, childhood hospitalizations, and parental arguments, all provide threats to our perception of nurturing. Thus virtually everyone has some abandonment feelings, perhaps locked deep in buried memories.

These feelings of inadequate nurturance lead to varying degrees of yearning to be loved and nurtured unconditionally, but always with the fear of rejection. Extremes of this feeling undoubtedly lead to attempts to please at virtually any cost, characteristic of those recently enshrined as "co-dependent."

Co-dependents have a pervasive sadness and in the most difficult of situations feel they can be happy only if they can receive the love they crave. Yet, unfortunately, perhaps because of conditioning from feeling rejected by their mother, such persons are almost magnetically attracted to a person, or goal, that is impossible to obtain. Undoubtedly such hopeless desire is the basis for a personality characterized by the psychiatrist Dr. Hans Eysenck as Type 1.[2]

Individuals who have Type 1 personality have an average life expectancy of 35 years less than Eysenck's Type 4. Approximately 75% of people who die of cancer have a lifelong Type 1 pattern. About 15% of those who die of heart disease are Type 1. A Type 1 individual who smokes has a 27% chance of developing cancer within 15 years of adulthood.

An even more serious deficit of nurturing, abuse in childhood, leads to lifelong anger. Physical, emotional, or sexual abuse can be equally damaging. Individuals who have a dominant feeling that their unhappiness was caused by abuse from someone are likely to be Eysenck's Type 2 personality. Approximately 75% of people who die of heart disease are Type 2. About 15% of those who die of cancer are Type 2.

Individuals who swing back and forth between anger and depression, between unfulfilled desire for a love that remains unattainable and unhappiness because of abuse, are Type 3. Approximately 9% of those who die of cancer or heart disease are Type 3. Type 3 persons live 7 years less than Type 4.

Type 4 individuals are those whom Eysenck calls "autonomous." These individuals either received superior nurturing in childhood or matured to recognize that *happiness is an inside job.* These are the individuals Maslowe called self-actualized. They realize that no one else can make them happy and no one can make them unhappy. These fortunate ones accept responsibility for choosing their overall attitude. They resolve past conflicts and hurts, give up unattainable yearnings, and forgive those who affronted or abused them. Life is for most individuals an attempt to reach Type 4 behavior.

In the teenage years nurturance encounters a special conflict— a need to give nurturing despite the continuing desire to be nurtured. Many of life's greatest dilemmas are the result of these apparently opposing needs. Only those who achieve Hans Selye's state of altruistic egotism move beyond the need to receive by learning that the ultimate feeling of nurturing is that of giving it unconditionally.[3]

Teenagers experience two other recurrent needs: freedom and sexuality. Freedom includes the need to make one's own decisions about every possible facet of life. Only those oppressed can properly appreciate the blessing of freedom to move, to speak, to vote, to pursue happiness.

Sexuality includes basic physiological and psychological urges, hormonally and environmentally conditioned, mixed ineffably with the desire to merge into another, to feel whole, to lose the feeling of separateness. Many have conceived of this feeling as the desire to return to God. In simple physical reality, sex is a drive toward the brief ecstasy of orgasm.

Wilhelm Reich believed that orgasm was an essential homeostatic mechanism and that anyone who failed to have an orgasm for three months would go insane.[4] If that were true, at one time or another most individuals would be insane. Nevertheless, repressed and/or ignored sexual needs undoubtedly account for many serious neurotic behaviors.

The Church, specifically, and the State in general have conspired to control people in a number of ways. Setting rules and laws governing sexual expression is a significant means of control. That which is essential has been so repressed that almost no one in Western society escapes the frustration of unfulfilled sexuality. The joyfulness of sexual expression is overlooked, even disclaimed from the pulpit to pornography.

Interestingly, even the most natural and harmless of sexual behaviors, self-stimulation, has been more attacked than any aspect of sexual activity. Reich, on the other hand, believed that no one could have a healthy, optimal sexual relation with another person unless he or she could please self well, first. For many individuals, probably most, true appreciation and exploration of personal satisfaction from self-stimulation is never even sought, let alone achieved!

Fear of abandonment, rejection or worse (according to the dictates of a particular religious belief), anger from abuse or suppression of freedom, and guilt over normal sexual nurturing desires then become the roots of a lifelong painful, often secret search for personal happiness.

Many individuals begin this search in the guise, often even to themselves, of pursuit of money, sexual conquests or submissions, or positions of power. These delusions of self-fulfillment are doomed to failure; for no activity, person, or other external factor, no matter how preoccupying, can satisfy the need to feel complete within oneself.

Actually, virtually all the problems of society are the result of attempts by the more aggressive seekers to fulfill their nurturing needs with the sex, money and/or power substitutes. Neurotic and psychotic behaviors revolve around attempts to achieve inner peace by more and more sex, money, or power. Thus billionaires, sexual philanderers, and dictators may still crave greater control. If control is their major motivation as a substitute for unmet, essential personal needs, ultimately they will fall. Ultimately life will seem abysmally empty, while materially full. They struggle hopelessly to survive while living in a constant state of alarm or fear of not having enough.

The will to live: a powerful drive to feel nurtured and satisfied, sustained by an unfaltering trust that somewhere usually "out there" is a place of complete peace, where one feels united with the universe, integrated with the whole. As long as one strives to feel "OK" through external acquisitions of sex, money, or power, pain and suffering result.

Fear, anxiety, anger, guilt, and depression—the roots of disease—may lead to one or more unresolved conflicts, including:

- Concerns about safety or survival.
- Fear of disasters.
- Sexual dysfunction or cravings.
- Fears about money or security.
- Poor self-esteem.
- Conflicts of responsibility.
- Interpersonal relationship problems.
- Inability to give, receive, or accept love.
- Inability to express needs or desires—conflicts of basic will.
- Confusion, unwise choices, or failure to accept intuitive knowing; inability to trust one's self.
- Spiritual crises.

The Internal Will—Insight

As we mature, we begin to recognize that pain, especially emotional pain, results often from a failure to accept things as they are; we desire external changes. This realization may lead to a major existential crisis, and even greater suffering. Or it may trigger a lifelong search to resolve the conflicts and to replace outward striving with inward security. Once the pain of realization comes, the seeker lusting after sex, money or power as fulfillment goals in life is never satisfied. One recognizes that internalized controls are the only avenues to self-empowerment.

So that the reader will clearly understand the difference, let us provide examples of internalized and externalized centers of control. Gwen grew up in a middle class family. She was extremely charming and cute as a child, and matured into adulthood as a beautiful woman. Her parents were excited about her potential for winning beauty contests, and gladly paid the fees and costs throughout childhood and her teen years. Gwen was also a cheerleader, football queen, and a clothing model during high school. Her parents cultivated "surface values"—image, comfort, material possessions—and fell short in providing a loving and warm home life built on the golden rule and empowering timeless values such as tolerance, generosity, joy, love, and respect. Gwen was perceived as an object of beauty, rather than a person of inner potential. By her late 20s Gwen's world was glamorous and bleak. She was a successful model, married to a wealthy man who was often away from home on business. She had all the external trappings of success that her parents had valued—a busy career based on her beauty, a financially secure marriage, and a showplace home—and a persistent empty feeling, unexplained loneliness, and increasing depression. She thought about having a baby to "give me something special," but she worried about the consequences of pregnancy to her figure and her husband's loving her. All her values about herself were based on how she reflected off others.

Contrast Gwen's dilemma with Jill's life. Jill too was raised in a middle-class family, and she too was charming and attractive from childhood. Hers was a loving family that from her birth was excited about her being part of their activities, and later, their decision-making. At age 2 she began drawing; they encouraged her obvious talent. They read to her, and discussed the contents of the story. They sang, traveled, and learned together. Jill was also the football queen in her senior year in high school, and editor of the yearbook. She was on the top of the honor role and was headed for college with plans to become a medical illustrator. She figured she could pick up some spending money there by modeling for a local department store a few hours a week, as she had done in high school.

The differences between Gwen and Jill were not externally obvious at the end of high school. They were both attractive, vibrant young women. In their late 20s, however, Gwen's dilemma was quickly obvious when contrasted with Jill's excitement about her career and goals, her achievements of substance to date which were leading her on "to possibilities I could never have imagined," she states in laughing wonder. Jill has internalized her values, and these have propelled her forward—her optimism, discipline, self-value. Gwen reaches inside and finds only emptiness, a lack of meaning for her life.

This internal control is unlikely in those who do not share the prevalent, primordial beliefs of all humanity, enumerated by one of the foremost psychiatrists of all time, Carl Jung, as:

- Belief in life after death (soul).
- Belief in God or universal power.
- Belief in the golden rule.[5]

Living the golden rule commits one to valuing not only one's self but others, to feeling needed, to setting meaningful goals, to serving and thus being fulfilled, striving to live the will of the soul, the source of one's ultimate growth potential.

As long as the conflicts remain unresolved, the body and mind suffer. Sooner or later physical or emotional dis-ease is likely. These manifestations of stress will probably affect the parts of the body symbolically associated with these primordial conflicts. For example, concerns of safety may affect our legs, our major mechanism for fight or flight. Sexual and financial insecurity and poor self-esteem affect our low back, pelvis, or sexual organs/functions. Interpersonal conflicts and those of responsibility affect our area of gut reaction—the solar plexus area. Love problems weaken the chest, breasts, and heart. Inability to express or communicate our needs and desires affects the mouth, throat, neck, thyroid, arms, or hands. Conflicts of wisdom, morality, or suppression of intuition may lead to brain or mind problems, defects of vision or hearing. Spiritual or existential crises lead to depression and/or unfocused anxiety.

If you suffer any pain or dysfunction in any part of your body or mind, you may wish to reflect further on the PRWL questionnaire which follows this discussion of the Transcendent Will.

The Transcendent Will

All of us desire the state of peace available to those who reach internal wisdom by recognizing that:

- I am responsible for my thoughts, feelings, and actions.
- I can choose my attitude towards every aspect of my life.
- I can change some internal and external factors.
- I can foster change in other people and situations, limited only by the wisdom of doing so (think about this carefully).
- For all aspects of life which I cannot change or choose not to fight—I am completely detached.
- I am not judgmental.
- I have no need to know why.
- With this realization optimally, internalized serenity prevails.

From the center of your being, in this state of harmony, you have a feeling of unconditional love—

- A desire to do good to yourself and to others.
- Striving becomes Being.

When living the Will of the Soul, all emotional yearning ceases, the idle chatter—the "chitta" of the mind as described by Patanjali—is quiet. The Dark Night of the Soul gives way to the Dawn of Enlightenment.

No other goal can accomplish so much. No other state can allow peace. Living the Transcendent Will is living the golden rule.

Quite simply, we have a responsibility to think and act in ways which are non-harmful; to use all forms of power wisely; and to love unconditionally—to help others and receive our nurturing through giving it freely and effortlessly.

To begin your journey and assess your unresolved needs, take the PRWL Test which follows on the next page.

Power—Responsibility—Wisdom—Love

Below are some items that you may accept or reject. Please indicate how you feel about each statement by placing a number from 0 to 3 in the spaces provided. A 0 indicates that you feel the statement is not at all true; 3 means that you feel the item is completely true. The following scale is to aid your understanding of the scoring system.

0 = Not at all true
1 = A little true
2 = Quite a bit true
3 = Completely true

1. **Issue: Security in the world at large.** I am concerned with:

a. Providing the necessities of life. _____

b. Feeling the world is safe (vs. threatening). _____

c. Feeling as though I "belong." _____

d. Feeling socially and financially supported in general. _____

Total these numbers. _____

2.a. **Issue: Sexuality.** I am concerned with:

1. Feeling adequate sexually. _____

2. Being my gender. _____

3. The level of my sexual activity. _____

4. Manipulation by others because
of race, color, sex, etc. _____

5. Feeling secure in my relationship with others. _____

Total these numbers. _____

b. **Issue: Financial Concerns:** I am concerned with:

1. Fear of poverty. _____

2. Feeling inadequate because of
   minimum financial power. _____

Total these numbers. _____

3. **Issue: Self-esteem,** a sense of personal power, feeling "OK"; feeling rejected or intimidated; surviving. I am concerned with:

a. A fear of being put down and intimidated. _____

b. A fear of assuming responsibility for myself, my

needs, commitments, finances, thoughts, etc. _____

c. Resentment over having to take responsibility for

someone else. _____

d. Anger from having power of choice violated. _____

e. Anger over being neglected or overlooked. _____

f. Being controlled by expectations of others. _____

Total these numbers. _____

4. **Issue: Love.** I am concerned with:

a Fear of not being loved. _____

b. Feeling unworthy of being loved. _____

c. Guilt over neglecting or rejecting others. _____

d. Feeling emotionally paralyzed by loneliness. _____

e. Harboring negative/judgmental feelings a lot. _____

f. Feeling unable to forgive. _____

g. Resentment over seeing others receive more love or attention. _____

h. Having abusive relationships. _____

i. Doing something or being with someone when my heart is not in it. _____

j. Having much grief and sorrow. _____

Total these numbers. _____

5. **Issue: Development of will power and personal expression.** I am concerned with:

a. Fear of self-assertion for my needs, feelings, opinions, desires. _____

b. Being dishonest to cover up my feelings or deny responsibility. _____

c. Using my will to control others. _____

d. My inability to say, "I"m sorry," "I love you,"

"I forgive you." _____

e. My inability to cry or express grief, hurt, sorrow ._____

Total these numbers. _____

6. **Issue: Using knowledge, wisdom, intuition.** I am concerned with:

a. My fear of self-examination, introspection. _____

b. Blocking my own intuition. _____

c. Misuse of my intellectual power; being deliberately deceptive. _____

d. Denying truth. _____

e. Believing I am intellectually inadequate. _____

f. My jealousy and insecurity over creative abilities of others. _____

g. My being closed to the value of other people's ideas. _____

h. Blaming others and repeating the same mistakes. _____

i. Being paranoid. _____

Total these numbers. _____

7. **Issue: Acceptance of life;** feeling fulfilled as though there is meaning in life. I am concerned with:

a Absence of faith, purpose, meaning. _____

b. Absence of faith and courage in myself. _____

c. Fear of really knowing myself. _____

d. Inability to see the larger pattern at work in my life. _____

e. Feeling that there is a soul, life after death, God. _____

Total these numbers. _____

Physical/Mental Health Scan
Now reflect on your past or current illnesses involving the related parts of your body. How strong is the lifelong health of:

- Your hips and legs.
- Your lower back, sexual organs, pelvis, and lower abdominal organs.

- Your upper abdomen, solar plexus, kidneys, liver, spleen, stomach, small intestine, transverse colon.
- Your chest, lungs, breasts, heart.
- Your neck, mouth, nose, throat, thyroid, parathryoid, arms, and hands.
- Your eyes, ears, brain, mind.
- Your sense of meaning in life—your faith that the purpose of life is good.

Return again and again to the PRWL Test and Physical/Mental Health Scan. They hold the key to insight and transcendence!

Notes—Chapter 8

1. Harris, Thomas A., *I'm OK, You're OK: A Practical Guide to Transactional Analysis* (New York: Harper-Rowe, 1969).

2. Eysenck, H.J., "Personality, Stress, and Cancer: Prediction and Prophylaxis," *British Journal of Medical Psychology* 61 (1988): 57–75.

3. Selye, Hans, *Stress Without Distress* (Philadelphia, PA: J.B. Lippincott Co., 1974).

4. Reich, Wilhelm. *Die Entdeckung des Orgons Erster Teil die Funktion des Orgasmus: Sexualokonomische Grundprobleme der Biologischen Energie.* (New York, NY: Farrar, Straus, & Giroux, Inc, 1968).

5. Jung, C.G., *Mysterium Coniunctionis: An Inquiry into the Separation and Synthesis of Psychic Opposites in Alchemy* (London: Routledge and Kegan Paul, 1963).

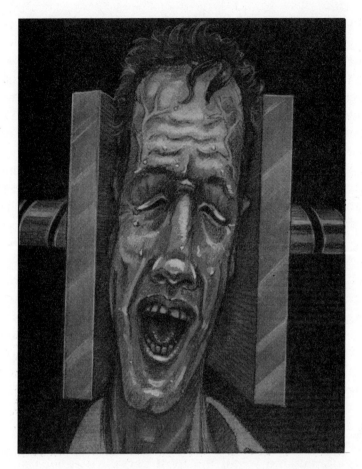

9

The Stress Connection

When you are sorrowful, look again in your heart, and you shall see that in truth you are weeping for that which has been your delight.

Dr. Hans Selye, the great Canadian researcher who developed the concept of the biological effects of stress, emphasized its ubiquity. Stress, positive and negative, pervades all life to the very cell. Our reactions to stress, largely determined by our genetic background and the early conditioning discussed in the last chapter, set the carburetor of our internal milieu.

On the other hand, many different external pressures can change the idling of our motor, revving it up or slowing it down. Joy, humor, and healthy exercise are positive stressors, creating beneficial reactions in our immune systems, neurochemicals, digestive process, and elsewhere, even in our relationships! On the negative side, we can be chemically, physically, or emotionally stressed to the point of mild to severely unhealthy symptoms or even death. Whenever any pressure becomes great enough to elicit an automatic *alarm* reaction, we experience stress. If we are well-attuned to feedback from our body, we may perceive subtle warnings that lead to changes in how much stress we continue to have. If we ignore the alarm signals and continue allowing the particular stress to recur on a regular basis, we *adapt*. But adapting to harmful stressors weakens us and lowers our tolerance or threshold for new stress. Increasing adaptation, even when we may not react to stressors with an outpouring of adrenalin, becomes a major contributor to wear and tear and is ultimately the cause of almost all illness.

Most stressors are not emotional, but are chemical, electromagnetic and physical. While their ability to elicit an alarm is specifically related to the quantity of that particular stress, your reaction will depend upon the total stress in your life at that given time— we all understand the meaning of "the last straw."

Chemical Stress

Throughout the world the most pervasive serious stress is tobacco use, or exposure to others' waste products of smoking. *Smoking, chewing, or sniffing of tobacco is responsible for almost half of all adult illness.* Admittedly, individuals may need to be "primed" by problems of nurturing to suffer the major consequences of smoking (chapter 8), but we seem to tolerate much more additional stress if we do not use tobacco products or become exposed to others' smoke. Furthermore, smokers' more common low self-esteem may make them more likely to smoke. Cancer of the lung and bladder, heart disease, emphysema, and sexual impotency are some of the major illnesses strikingly more prevalent with smokers. Even early excessive wrinkling is unequivocally aggravated by smoking.

The number two chemical stress, in terms of illness, is related to the use of alcohol. Alcohol is responsible for more teenage deaths than any other single factor because of accidents created by alcoholics. Cirrhosis, accidents, child and spouse abuse, and resultant emotional trauma are the major illnesses of alcohol. Even "moderate" alcohol is associated with premature birth, congenital malformations, and accelerated memory loss with aging.

Of the commonly used chemical stressors, none equals the harmful and costly impact of tobacco and alcohol. Nevertheless, "pop" is certainly right up there in popularity, consumed by Americans at the rate of a gallon per week per person. Loaded with sugar, caffeine, and phosphate of soda, pop interferes with calcium and magnesium metabolism and aggravates or causes osteoporosis, the single most common cause of premature death in the elderly, because of fractured hips! Pop consumption can aggravate obesity, diabetes, high blood pressure, and heart disease (through magnesium deficiency).

The caffeine in coffee and tea becomes a stressor when a person consumes more than four cups per day. Water-extracted decaffeinated coffee is probably safe in any usual amount, though some health authorities dispute that consumers can help themselves in these decisions by tuning into their bodies and listening to the messages. Each person's metabolism and nutritional needs are unique to some extent.

While sugar, in moderation, is probably not harmful, Americans consume more sugar per capita than any other people in the world, *more than 125 pounds* per year per person. Cancer of the colon, diabetes, obesity, heart disease, and osteoporosis are all influenced by excess sugar. Twenty teaspoons of sugar block your white blood cells' ability to eat bacteria by 95% for well over four hours! One "fast food" milk shake contains 20 to 25 teaspoons of sugar.

Salt is a stressor for those who pour it on. The average American consumes over four times the optimal amount, optimal being about a half teaspoon per day. Two to five teaspoons daily aggravate high blood pressure, contributing ultimately to strokes.

Besides these common social chemicals, there are hundreds of thousands of chemicals released into the soil, water, and air that are often undetectable by the senses. The total of these chemicals cannot be adequately measured, but cancer and allergies are undoubtedly increased significantly by exposure to general pollution.

Ignorance is the failure to accept the truth when it is presented. Be aware that the measurable and controllable chemical stressors are responsible for a majority of deaths, illnesses, and common problems such as insomnia, depression, and irritability. If you value your health, avoid tobacco, stay away from illegal drugs, do not use medications carelessly, and at least minimize your consumption of alcohol, caffeine, sugar, pop, and salt. These choices of a healthier lifestyle cut your illness rate by more than 50%, allowing you to feel better, think more clearly, and be less stressed out by the common psychological wear and tear of daily life.

Nutrition is such an important aspect of health that it will be covered separately later in this chapter.

Physical Stress.

In the last 70 years, most Americans have become "couch potatoes," seated in a chair or snuggled on a couch, often indoors, in front of a television screen where advertising pushes and features the unhealthy lifestyle. So what is wrong here? The sedentary lifestyle contributes significantly to obesity, tension headaches, malnutrition, and degenerative diseases.

The body is a motion machine. When it is insufficiently physically active, it declines in function as it accumulates the wounds of physical inactivity. The body needs natural light and clean air to work best.

Consider the typical American workplace—managed air, unopenable windows, sedentary occupations—and a home life with many of these same ingredients. Actually, stress is commonly known to elicit a *fight or flight* response. Thus the *normal* response to stress is physical; and adequate exercise is the single best antidote for non-avoidable stress. Lack of physical exercise is a major contributor to heart attacks, obesity, depression, and fatigue, as well as to increasing stiffness and aching as we age.

Inadequate use of the body machine ironically leads to trauma or accidents; 80% of the time these are the result of care-less-ness, often brought on by anger or anxiety, sometimes hurting others in the process. The only preventive measure for such accidents is to keep your body healthy and your intuition active at all times (more about enhancing intuition later).

Most other physical stressors, such as changes in barometric pressure, are not easily avoidable. Increasingly, however, we learn that electromagnetic pollution may be a major contributor to birth defects, miscarriage, cancer, and possible other problems such as chronic fatigue. Avoid electric blankets and heated waterbeds. Cover the latter with a heat reflector and sheepskin and save electricity as well as pollution. Keep electrical gadgets, such as radios and clocks, three feet or more away from your body. If you work on a computer, have it checked for electromagnetic fields. Don't stand in front of microwaves. Sit six feet or more away from television sets.

Avoiding some infections is just a matter of common sense. Wash your hands after using the toilet. Be sure milk, water, and food are free of contamination. Don't take illegal or unnecessary drugs, never "share" needles, avoid sex with strangers, and avoid anal sex; all of these are major sources of the AIDS virus.

Get fresh air and natural light as much as is possible. If you work indoors, try to have fresh air and full-spectrum fluorescent light. If you live in a big city or in highly polluted air, I recommend Alpine Aire™ air filters. They appear to do a better job than half a dozen other air filters I've tried.

Emotional Stress

The roots of emotional stress were discussed in chapter 8. Chemical and physical stressors are major aggravators of an already fragile system.

Ultimately, emotional stress is the result of fear of the Big Five: Death, Illness, Financial Insecurity, Abandonment, or a crisis regarding Moral Values. Recognizing that one's reactions to fear are the result of one or more of these five threats is often a great help. Begin the process of identifying your sources of distress by being aware of your fears related to the Big Five. Then ask yourself:

- Am I anxious because I fear death, illness, poverty or deprivation, loss of love, moral conflict, or meaning in life (purpose for existing)?
- Am I angry because of injustice related to any of these five factors?
- Do I feel guilty because I feel I haven't lived up to my expectations?

- Can I feel better by being upset?
- Can I solve any of these problems by:
  1. *Asserting Myself?*
     - Arguing?
     - Stating my point of view clearly, energetically?
     - Fighting?
     - Taking legal action?
  2. *Fleeing?*
     - If I cannot solve the problem or correct it, can I divorce it with joy because I don't have to put up with it any more?
  3. *Forgiving?*
     - If I cannot change the problem or divorce it, am I willing to accept and forgive just for personal peace?
     - Who suffers if I continue to be upset?
     - Am I willing to take responsibility for my reactions, to use wisdom, to be open to possible alternate solutions, to make choices, to exert my personal power, and to love myself adequately to resolve these concerns?

Reflect upon these questions often. If you still cannot resolve your distress, you will find a number of experiential opportunities to gain insight and detachment later in this book.

For an overall review of your total life stress and its effects upon your health, take the **Personal Stress Assessment Test** beginning on page 117 and see just how Health-Wise you are.

Most people recognize stress as a contributor to some illnesses. Actually, stress is the single greatest cause of illness; from the common cold to cancer, stress aggravates or causes disease and reduces the quality of life.

To understand stress adequately, you need to know that stress is *relative*—that is, except for identical twins, the level of stress tolerance varies tremendously among individuals. To some extent, the stress reaction is the result of attitude: if you consider a glass half full, you are not likely to be stressed; if you think of the glass as half empty, you are more likely to feel stress.

More importantly, Total Life Stress is the result of all the pressure in your life:
Chemical
Physical
Emotional/Attitudinal

The Stress Triangle

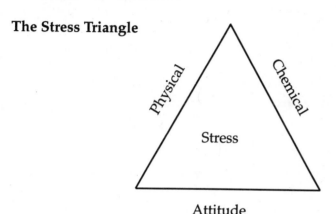

Ultimately, it is your *attitude* that determines your habits and your reactions to events in your life.

Major stressors (in order of importance in each category):

Chemical	Physical	Emotional
Nicotine	Inactivity	Fear which leads to:
Alcohol	Accidents	Anxiety
Excess Calories	Excess Calories	Anger
Pollution	Physical Work While	Guilt
Sugar	in Poor Condition	Depression
Caffeine	Infectious Agents	
Drugs	Electromagnetic	
Salt		

The good news is that most stress is controllable. First you must recognize what is stressing you; then you can begin to do something about stress in your life.

Stresses (Lifestyle) Associated with the Most Common Specific Diseases

Here is a sample of the dominant stressors in some of the most common illnesses.

High Blood Pressure
1. Salt Intake
2. Cigarette Smoking
3. Obesity
4. Caffeine
5. Physical Activity
6. Diabetes
7. Low Fiber Diet
8. Emotional Stress

Diabetes
1. Sugar
2. Obesity
3. Low fiber diet
4. Physical inactivity
5. Caffeine
6. Heredity
7. Excess total stress (emotional crises, etc.)

Cancer of Breast
1. Low fiber diet
2. High fat diet
3. Caffeine (?)
4. Depression

Cancer of Colon
1. Low fiber diet
2. High fat diet
3. Depression

Cancer of Lung
1. Cigarette smoking
2. Depression

Coronary Artery Disease (Heart Attacks)
1. Cigarette smoking
2. Low fiber diet
3. High fat diet
4. Emotional stress
5. Obesity
6. High blood pressure
7. Caffeine
8. Diabetes
9. Physical inactivity
10. Heredity
11. Anger

Strokes
1. High blood pressure (One might include the subcategories of high blood pressure as well)

Appendicitis, Diverticulitis and Diverticulosis, Gall Stones, Varicose Veins, Hemorrhoids
1. Low fiber diet
2. High fat diet
3. High sugar diet

Now take the Total Life Stress Test and begin to see what you need to do to reduce stress in your life.

Personal Stress Assessment
Total Life Stress Test

Name _____

Date _____

Record your stress points on the lines in the right-hand margin, and indicate subtotals in the boxes at the end of each section. Then add your subtotals to determine your total score

I. CHEMICAL STRESS

A. Dietary Stress

<u>Average Daily Sugar Consumption</u>

Sugar added to food or drink	1 point per 5 teaspoons	_____
Sweet roll, piece of pie/cake, brownie, other dessert	1 point each	_____
Coke or can of pop, candy bar	2 points each	_____
Banana split, commercial milk shake, sundae, etc.	5 points each	_____
White flour (white bread, spaghetti, etc.)	5 points	_____

<u>Average Daily Salt Consumption</u>

Little or no "added" salt	0 points	_____
Few salty foods (pretzels, potato chips, etc.)	0 points	_____

Moderate "added" salt and/or salty foods at least once per day	3 points	_____
Heavy salt user, regularly (use of "table salt" and/or salty foods at least twice per day)	10 points	_____

Average Daily Caffeine Consumption

Coffee	1/2 point each	_____
Tea	1/2 point each	_____
Cola Drink or Mountain Dew®	1 point each cup	_____
2 Anacin® or APC tabs	1/2 point each	_____
Caffeine Benzoate tablets (NoDoz,® Vivarin,® etc.)	2 points each	_____
	Dietary Subtotal	_____

B. Other Chemical Stress

Drinking Water

Chlorinated only	1 point	_____
Chlorinated and fluoridated	2 points	_____

Soil and Air Pollution

Live within 10 miles of city of 500,000 or more	10 points	_____
Live within 10 miles of city of 250,000 or more	5 points	_____

Live within 10 miles of city of 50,000 or more	2 points	_____
Live in the country but use pesticides, herbicides, and/or chemical fertilizer	10 points	_____
Exposed to cigarette smoke of someone else more than one hour per day	5 points	_____

Drugs (any amount of usage)

Antidepressants	1 point	_____
Tranquilizers	3 points	_____
Sleeping pills	3 points	_____
Narcotics	5 points	_____
Other pain relievers	3 points	_____

Nicotine

3–10 cigarettes per day	5 points	_____
11–20 cigarettes per day	15 points	_____
21–30 cigarettes per day	20 points	_____
31–40 cigarettes per day	35 points	_____
Over 40 cigarettes per day	40 points	_____
Cigar(s) per day	1 point each	_____
Pipeful(s) of tobacco per day	1 point each	_____
Chewing tobacco—"chews" per day	1 point each	_____

Average Daily Alcohol Consumption

1 oz. whiskey, gin, vodka, etc.	2 points each	_____
8 oz. beer	2 points each	_____
4-6 oz. glass of wine	2 points each	_____

Other Chemical Subtotal_____

Chemical Total _____

II. PHYSICAL STRESS

Weight

Underweight more than 10 lbs.	5 points	_____
10 to 15 lbs. overweight	5 points	_____
16 to 25 lbs. overweight	10 points	_____
26 to 40 lbs. overweight	25 points	_____
More than 40 pounds overweight	40 points	_____

Activity

Adequate exercise,* 3 days or more per week	0 points	_____
Some physical exercise, 1 or 2 days per week	15 points	_____
No regular exercise	40 points	_____

*Adequate means doubling heartbeat and/or sweating a minimum of 30 minutes per time.

Work Stress

Sit most of the day	3 points	_____
Industrial/factory worker	3 points	_____
Overnight travel more than once a week	5 points	_____
Work more than 50 hours per week	2 points per hour over 50	_____
Work varying shifts	10 points	_____
Work night shift	5 points	_____
Heavy labor—physically fit	0 points	_____
Heavy labor—not physically fit	40 points	_____
	Physical Total	_____

III. ATTITUDINAL STRESS

A. Holmes-Rahe Social Readjustment Rating*
(Circle the mean values that correspond with life events listed below which you have experienced the past 12 months.)

Death of a spouse	100
Divorce	73
Marital separation	65

*See Holmes, T.H. and R. H. Rahe, "The Social Readjustment Rating Scale," *Journal of Psychosomatic Research* 11 (1967): 213–218, for complete wording of these items. Reproduced with permission of the authors and publisher.

Jail term	63
Death of a close family member	63
Personal injury or illness	53
Marriage	50
Fired at work	47
Marital reconciliation	45
Retirement	45
Change in health of family member	44
Pregnancy	40
Sexual difficulties	39
Gain of new family member	39
Business readjustment	39
Change in financial state	38
Death of close friend	37
Change to different line of work	36
Change in number of arguments with spouse	35
Mortgage over $20,000	31
Foreclosure of mortgage or loan	30
Change in responsibilities at work	29
Son or daughter leaving home	29
Trouble with in-laws	29
Outstanding personal achievement	28
Spouse beginning or stopping work	26
Beginning or ending school	25
Change in living conditions	24
Revision of personal habits	23
Trouble with boss	20
Change in work hours or conditions	20
Change in residence	20
Change in schools	19

Change in recreation	19
Change in church activities	18
Change in social activities	17
Mortgage or loan less than $20,000	16
Change in sleeping habits	15
Change in eating habits	15
Vacation, especially if away from home	13
Christmas, or other major holiday stress	12
Minor violations of the law	11

(Add the mean values to get the Holmes Rahe total. Then refer to the conversion table to determine your number of stress points.)

Conversion Table

Your number of points:	Holmes-Rahe less than	Your number of points:	Holmes-Rahe less than
0	60	16	280
1	110	17	285
2	160	18	290
3	170	19	295
4	180	20	300
5	190	21	305
6	200	22	310
7	210	23	315
8	220	24	320
9	230	25	325
10	240	26	330
11	250	27	335
12	260	28	340
13	265	29	345
14	270	30	350
15	275	Anything over 351 = 40 +	

Holmes-Rahe Social Readjustment Rating (Converted) _____

B. Other Emotional Stress

Sleep

Less than 7 hours per night	3 points	_____
Usually 7 or 8 hours per night	0 points	_____
More than 8 hours per night	2 points	_____

Relaxation

Relax only during sleep	10 points	_____
Relax or meditate at least 20 minutes per day	0 points	_____

Frustration at work

Enjoy work	0 points	_____
Mildly frustrated by job	1 point	_____
Moderately frustrated by job	3 points	_____
Very frustrated by job	5 points	_____
Lack of authority at job	5 points	_____
Boss doesn't trust me	5 points	_____

Marital Status

Married, happily	0 points	_____
Married, moderately unhappy	2 points	_____

Married, very unhappy	5 points	_____
Unmarried man over 30	5 points	_____
Unmarried woman over 30	2 points	_____

Usual Mood

Happy, well adjusted	0 points	_____
Moderately angry, depressed or frustrated	10 points	_____
Very Angry, depressed, or frustrated	20 points	_____

Overall Attitude

Hopeless	10-40 points	_____
Depressed	10-40 points	_____
Unable to achieve major goal	10-40 points	_____
Unable to achieve close love/ intimacy	10-40 points	_____
Frustrated, annoyed, and/or angry because someone attacked or harmed me or prevented me from happiness	10-40 points	_____
Satisfied and in control of my life	0 points	_____
Experience happiness regularly	0 points	_____
Believe I am responsible for my happiness	0 points	_____

Believe and experience happiness
  is an inside job   0 points   ____
Any Other Major Emotional Stress Not
  Mentioned Above.
  You Judge Intensity.   10-40 points   ____

Attitudinal Total ____

TOTAL LIFE STRESS

I. Chemical Total   _____

II. Physical Total   _____

III. Attitudinal Total   _____

TLS Total   _____

If your score exceeds 24 points, you probably will feel better if you reduce your stress; greater than 50 points, you definitely need to eliminate stress in your life.

Circle your stressor with the highest number of points and work first to eliminate it; then circle your next greatest stressor, overcome it; and so on.

Now look at some of the ways your body may react to stress. Please be aware, if you have any major/worrisome symptom, or more than 15 total symptoms, you should consult your physician before deciding that stress is the cause of your symptoms.

Possible Stress Symptoms
For the following questions, please indicate YES or NO. YES means *now*, or in the **past 12 months.**

YES NO

___ ___   1. Do you have headaches more than once a week?

___ ___   2. Do you have either a repeated buzzing or other noises in your ears?

___ ___ 3. Do you get motion sickness by riding in either a car or plane?

___ ___ 4. Is your throat ever sore when you don't have a cold?

___ ___ 5. Do you ever get either pains or tightness in your chest?

___ ___ 6. Are you troubled by heartburn?

___ ___ 7. Do you suffer discomfort in the pit of your stomach?

___ ___ 8. Do you easily become nauseated (feel like vomiting)?

___ ___ 9. Have you either gained or lost much weight recently?

___ ___ 10. Have you lost your interest in eating lately?

___ ___ 11. Do you always seem to be hungry?

___ ___ 12. Do you urinate more than five or six times per day?

___ ___ 13. Do you have a constant feeling that you have to urinate?

___ ___ 14. Are you troubled by diarrhea?

___ ___ 15. Do you bite your nails?

___ ___ 16. Are you troubled by stuttering or stammering?

___ ___ 17. Are you a sleep walker?

___ ___ 18. Do you suffer from nervous exhaustion?

___ ___ 19. Are you frequently ill?

___ ___ 20. Are you a sickly person?

___ ___ 21. Are you troubled by pains in the back or shoulders?

___ ___ 22. Does your skin either itch or burn?

___ ___ 23. Do you have trouble with either dizziness or light-headedness?

___ ___ 24. Do you have either cold hands and/or feet even in hot weather?

_____ _____ 25. Do you have a tendency either to shake or to tremble?

_____ _____ 26. Do you sweat a lot?

_____ _____ 27. Do you have hot flashes?

_____ _____ 28. Does every little effort leave you short of breath?

_____ _____ 29. Do you seem to feel exhausted or fatigued most of the time?

_____ _____ 30. Do you have difficulty either falling or staying asleep?

_____ _____ 31. Do you fail to get the exercise you should?

_____ _____ 32. Are you definitely overweight?

_____ _____ 33. Are you definitely underweight?

_____ _____ 34. Do you usually eat between meals (sweets and other foods)?

_____ _____ 35. Do you often have small accidents or injuries?

_____ _____ 36. Is it usually hard for you to make up your mind?

_____ _____ 37. Are you usually either unhappy or depressed?

_____ _____ 38. Do you cry often?

_____ _____ 39. Does your life look entirely hopeless?

_____ _____ 40. Does worrying often get you down?

_____ _____ 41. Are you either extremely shy or sensitive?

_____ _____ 42. Does criticism usually upset you?

_____ _____ 43. Do little annoyances either get on your nerves or make you angry?

_____ _____ 44. Do you flare up in anger if you can't have what you want right away?

_____ _____ 45. Are you nervous around strangers?

_____ _____ 46. Do you find it hard to make decisions?

_____ _____ 47. Do you find it hard either to concentrate or to remember?

___ ___ 48. Do you often feel lonely?

___ ___ 49. Do you have difficulty relaxing?

___ ___ 50. Are you troubled by either frightening dreams or frightening thoughts?

___ ___ 51. Have you considered committing suicide?

___ ___ 52. Are you disturbed by either work or family problems?

___ ___ 53. Have you desired psychiatric help?

___ ___ 54. Are you often or usually tense and uptight?

___ ___ 55. Are you often nervous or jittery?

___ ___ 56. Are you easily upset?

___ ___ 57. Are you in low spirits most of the time?

___ ___ 58. Are you often in very low spirits?

___ ___ 59. Do you believe that your life is out of your hands and controlled by external factors?

___ ___ 60. Is your life empty, filled only with despair?

___ ___ 61. In your life, do you have no goals or aims at all?

___ ___ 62. Have you completely failed to progress toward your life goals?

___ ___ 63. Concerning your freedom to make your own choices, do you believe you are completely bound by limitations of heredity and environment?

___ ___ 64. Is your urine stream either very weak or very slow?

___ ___ 65. Do you have trouble having erections?

___ ___ 66. Do you have premature ejaculation?

___ ___ 67. Are you having trouble with your menstrual periods?

___ ___ 68. Do you feel either bloated or irritable before your periods?

___ ___ 69. Are you often either weak or sick with your periods?

___ ___ 70. Do you often have to lie down when your periods start?

___ ___ 71. Are you usually tense and jumpy with your periods?

___ ___ 72. Do you have constant severe hot flashes and sweats?

___ ___ 73. Do you experience jaw clenching or pain?

___ ___ 74. Do you grind your teeth?

___ ___ 75. Do you experience frequent blushing?

___ ___ 76. Do you experience a dry mouth?

___ ___ 77. Do you have trouble swallowing?

___ ___ 78. Do you have allergies?

___ ___ 79. Do you experience constipation?

___ ___ 80. Do you experience attacks of panic?

___ ___ 81. Do you have a decreased sexual desire?

___ ___ 82. Do you have an inability to have orgasm?

___ ___ 83. Do you have nightmares?

___ ___ 84. Do you have problems with friends?

___ ___ 85. Do you have problems at work?

___ ___ 86. Do you experience obsessive thinking?

Although any of the above symptoms could also be part of more serious problems, the following are symptoms which unequivocally should be checked by your physician before you try stress reduction.

See Your Doctor Symptoms

___ 1. Have you had either lumps or swelling in your neck?

___ 2. Does your eyesight blur?

___ 3. Is your eyesight getting worse?

___ 4. Do you ever see double?

_____ 5. Do you ever see colored halos around lights?

_____ 6. Do your eyes either blink or water most of the time?

_____ 7. Have you experienced loss of vision?

_____ 8. Have you had difficulty hearing?

_____ 9. Have you had any earaches lately?

_____ 10. Have you been troubled by running ears lately?

_____ 11. Do you have any sore swellings on either your gums or your jaws?

_____ 12. Is your tongue either sore or sensitive?

_____ 13. Have your taste senses changed lately?

_____ 14. Is your nose stuffed up when you don't have a cold?

_____ 15. Does your nose run when you don't have a cold?

_____ 16. Do you have frequent sneezing spells?

_____ 17. Have you ever had head colds two or more months in a row?

_____ 18. Does your nose bleed for no reason at all?

_____ 19. Is your voice hoarse when you don't have a cold?

_____ 20. Is it either difficult or painful for you to swallow?

_____ 21. Do you either wheeze or have to gasp to breathe?

_____ 22. Are you bothered by coughing spells?

_____ 23. Do you cough up a lot of phlegm (thick spit)?

_____ 24. Have you coughed up blood?

_____ 25. Do you get chest colds more than once a month?

_____ 26. Have you been told that you have high blood pressure?

_____ 27. Have you been told that you have low blood pressure?

_____ 28. Have you been told you have heart trouble?

_____ 29. Have you been bothered by either a thumping or racing heart?

_____ 30. Do you awaken at night short of breath?

_____ 31. Do you get short of breath just sitting?

_____ 32. Do you feel bloated after eating?

_____ 33. Are you troubled by belching?

_____ 34. Have you vomited blood?

_____ 35. Have you had an ulcer?

_____ 36. Do you frequently get up at night to urinate?

_____ 37. Do you either wet your pants or wet the bed?

_____ 38. Have you had either burning or pains when you urinate?

_____ 39. Has your urine been either brown, black, or bloody?

_____ 40. Do you have great difficulty starting your urine?

_____ 41. Are you constipated more than twice a month?

_____ 42. Are your bowel movements ever either black or bloody?

_____ 43. Are your bowel movements ever grey in color?

_____ 44. Do you suffer pains when you move your bowels?

_____ 45. Have you had any bleeding from your rectum?

_____ 46. Do severe stomach pains double you up?

_____ 47. Do you have frequent stomach trouble?

_____ 48. Have you had intestinal worms?

_____ 49. Has a diagnosis of hemorrhoids (piles) been made?

_____ 50. Have you had jaundice (yellow eyes and skin)?

_____ 51. Have you had any serious problems with your genitals (privates)?

_____ 52. Do you have a hernia (rupture)?

_____ 53. Do you have either kidney or bladder disease?

_____ 54. Are you frequently confined to bed by illness?

_____ 55. Are you troubled with either stiff or painful muscles or joints?

_____ 56. Are your joints ever swollen?

_____ 57. Are your feet often painful?

_____ 58. Are there any swellings in either your armpits or groin?

_____ 59. Do you have trouble with either swollen feet or ankles?

_____ 60. Are you getting cramps in your legs at night or upon walking?

_____ 61. Do you have trouble stopping even a small cut from bleeding?

_____ 62. Do you bruise easily?

_____ 63. Do you ever either faint or feel faint?

_____ 64. Is any part of your body always numb?

_____ 65. Has any part of your body been paralyzed?

_____ 66. Have you blacked out?

_____ 67. Have you had either fits or convulsions?

_____ 68. Do you have a tendency to be either too hot or too cold?

_____ 69. Do you have bleeding gums?

_____ 70. Is your tongue often badly coated?

_____ 71. Do you have varicose veins (swollen veins) in your legs?

_____ 72. Has a doctor told you that you have prostate trouble?

_____ 73. Have you had either burning or any unusual discharge from your penis?

_____ 74. Are there either any swellings or lumps on your testicles?

_____ 75. Do your testicles get painful?

_____ 76. Have you had bleeding between your periods?

_____ 77. Do you have heavy bleeding with your periods?

_____ 78. Have you taken any birth control pills?

_____ 79. Have you ever had any lumps in your breasts?

____ 80. Have you had any excess discharges from your vagina?

____ 81. Have you had any major unexplained pain?

____ 82. Have you had any rapid weight loss without dieting?

____ 83. Have you had any problem that worries you?

If you have 15 or more of the "Possible Stress Symptoms" or any of the "See Your Doctor Symptoms," you should have a thorough checkup by your physician. If he or she tells you it is all in your head, or "just nerves," then it is reasonable to use the Shealy Stress Control System.™

Escaping Nutritional Stress

Nutrition has received more public and less scientific attention than any other important health issue. Even more unfortunately, much of the research has been directed at one, and only one, aspect of nutrition: fat. In the early 1950s it became apparent that cholesterol is a major contributor to atherosclerosis, especially heart attacks. This preoccupation has led to ignoring a growing number of important facts, a few examples follow:

- Eggs do not "raise" blood cholesterol levels in most people.
- Butter is a much higher quality food than margarine because of the artificially hydrogenated fats in margarine.
- Stress raises cholesterol much more than does diet.
- Lowering fat excessively leads to dangerously low HDL cholesterol, the "good" aspect of cholesterol, in some people.
- Food *combinations* affect body weight and cholesterol more than absolute fat intake.
- Physical exercise lowers cholesterol and raises HDL better than dietary restriction and has many added health benefits.
- "Primitive" diets, such as the native Eskimo diet, very high in fat but low in carbohydrate, do not lead to high cholesterol.

Given facts like these, we can easily understand the confusion people commonly feel about nutrition. Furthermore, there is much evidence that our soils are highly deficient in some essential nutrients; the U.S.D.A.'s measurements of the nutrient content of foods were mostly done 35 to 40 years ago. Today huge quantities of our food, both "fresh" and processed, are imported from all over the world, often harvested prematurely, stored for long periods of time (thanks to the increased use of preservatives), and contaminated with pesticides and herbicides in order to increase shelf life. Highly processed food typically loses nutrient value. This includes "fast food," which often is prepared in reused fat and is loaded with salt, sugar, and added chemicals.

In general, my advice is simple: Eat a wide variety of real food (that is, previously unprocessed), grown as near you as possible. Some of the greatest opportunities for financial success and benefits to health lie in small acreage farming, growing foods organically within 25 miles of cities. If possible, find a farmer near you to obtain as much of your food as possible.

Additional nutritional ideas may be helpful from these sources:

- The American Heart Association protocol
- The Macrobiotic, McDougall, or Pritikin protocol
- The Broda Barnes protocol

The American Heart Association (AHA)

This approach is middle-of-the-road, much better than the average American diet. I disagree with it on only one major point—do not use margarine. If you wish to use a "spread," mix butter half and half with olive or safflower oil—much better for you than margarine. Or use light cream cheese—it has less fat than margarine and tastes better. You can even make a fat-free cream cheese by pouring nonfat yogurt into a coffee filter, letting it sit in the refrigerator overnight, and use as is or mix with Butter Buds®. You can also use Butter Buds® to flavor vegetables, potatoes, and rice and avoid all fat.

Otherwise, the AHA diet calls for limiting eggs to about four per week; using skimmed milk; limiting meats, especially red meats; avoiding fried foods; minimizing fats and oils; eating lots of whole grains and vegetables. Overall this diet provides calories at a level of 30% fat, about 15% protein, and 55% carbohydrate. It is much better than the 45% fat consumed by most Americans.

The Macrobiotic, McDougall, or Pritikin

The lean cuisine of Pritikin, McDougall, and macrobiotic further restricts fat to about 10%, with 10% protein and 80% carbohydrate. They all urge avoiding fatty meats, especially red meats; using virtually no added fats or oils; emphasizing vegetables and grains. McDougall is totally vegetarian. And none of these diets tastes as good as the AHA or Barnes diets. They do lower cholesterol in most people, but may lower HDL. Additionally, those people who are "fast oxidizers," as defined by Watson,[1] will likely feel starved by these diets much of the time. For "slow oxidizers" these three diets are probably ideal.

The Broda Barnes Diet

Based on his work with over 10,000 patients, Dr. Broda Barnes, a physician and physiologist, reported that the ideal diet for most people is one with approximately 20% protein, 15% carbohydrate, and 65% fat—any kind of fat.[2] And he published numerous papers to prove his point. Unfortunately, his work has been largely ignored and never extensively studied by anyone else. My intuition says his diet is excellent for fast oxidizers but should be used very carefully by anyone with already existing atherosclerosis or heart disease. Similarly my intuition does not allow me to recommend using thyroid medication in virtually everyone. Thus, I offer this diet as an alternative for those who wish to try it, recognizing I have not followed Dr. Barnes all the way!

The essential factors of the Barnes diet are to avoid grains, legumes, potatoes, starches, sugars, and high sugar-content fruits. Beyond those restrictions you eat unlimited vegetables, moderate amounts of any kind of meat, use large amounts of fatty salad dressings, and drink moderate amounts of whole milk. You can have up to three citrus fruits or servings of melon or strawberries per day.

This diet provides remarkably good flavor; slow, gradual

return of hunger; and for many people, weight loss. It appears many may lower cholesterol by eating this diet, which uses fat for fuel instead of carbohydrate. It leads to much less intestinal gas and probably "works" by increasing excretion of bile to release cholesterol.

If you decide to try the Barnes approach, you must have your cholesterol, HDL cholesterol, and triglycerides checked first and again at one month, three months, six months, and at least annually thereafter. Very few physicians will support a decision to try this diet because it has received little attention from the medical "establishment." Until more data is in, however, it is a possible alternative, especially for fast oxidizers who exercise adequately.

For those individuals with really high cholesterol, strong family histories of heart disease, and already known atherosclerosis, I recommend first trying a lean cuisine diet. If that doesn't work, along with optimal physical exercise and relaxation, try first niacin, timed release, four per day. If that doesn't work, try lean cuisine plus two tablespoons flax seed oil per day. Vegetable sterols sold as "cholestratin" may also help. All drugs carry some risks and should be a last resort.

There is one other possibility: Use a Barnes-type breakfast and a lean cuisine lunch and dinner. You would wind up with approximately the same ratios recommended by the American Heart Association and have a marvelous tasting breakfast which lasts well.

But if you are going to play with any of these dietary approaches, monitor your blood fats as indicated above and your general feeling of well-being and energy.

For those individuals who are depressed, I recommend having an essential amino acid profile done by blood testing and a magnesium load test. Virtually 100% of depressed patients are deficient in one or more essential amino acids, the building blocks for many neurochemicals which influence mood; 100% are deficient in magnesium.

For those with high blood pressure, chronic fatigue, panic attacks, heart attack, irregular heart rhythm, and osteoporosis, I consider a magnesium load test essential. If you have a heart attack and do not receive a shot of magnesium, your chances of dying are 70% greater! Magnesium deficiency is best treated with daily shots of magnesium intravenously for 6-12 days plus oral magnesium forever afterwards. Magnesium taurate, 500 mg two or three times a day, is the oral supplement of choice. Only people with kidney failure need worry about getting too much magnesium. Seventy percent of men and 80% of women take in inadequate amounts of magnesium.

Foods highest in magnesium include carrots, peanuts, sesame seeds, and beets. But you would need to eat 17 tablespoons of peanut butter to get your daily requirement of magnesium.

Other than magnesium, considering the poor quality of many foods, I recommend the following routine supplements daily:

- B-Complex, 25 to 100 mg
- Beta Carotene, 25,000 units
- Vitamin C, 2 grams
- Vitamin E, 400 units

For those with allergies, try:

- Vitamin C, 5 to 15 grams, if your intestines tolerate it.
- Beta Carotene, 200,000 units
- B-Complex, 100 mg
- Vitamin E, 400 units

Actually, according to government statistics, since at least 1960, Americans have averaged significant deficits in intake of calcium, magnesium, Vitamin B6, Vitamin E, and zinc, with increasing excesses of phosphorous, which would aggravate calcium and magnesium deficiencies.[3]

Finally, there is the question of good and adequate water. Ideally you need a minimum of one and a half quarts per day and up to two and a half quarts. Most city water is loaded with chlorine and fluoride, tastes awful, and often has weak concentrations of carcinogenic agents. Much farm water is contaminated. Distilled water tastes flat, may deplete you of calcium and magnesium, and is expensive. Bottled spring water is usually good but expensive. The simplest alternative is filtered water. You can buy a good water filter inexpensively and it does a good job of removing most contaminants. I think the Aqua Pure™ is an excellent device. We use it at our clinic.

Most herb teas taste good and provide a good source for water. If you really don't like water, try a few drops of lime juice or Rose's lime juice in a quart of water. The usual recommendation of six to eight glasses (8 oz.) a day is excellent. If you weigh more than 110 pounds, make it eight glasses; and if you're over 150 pounds, go to 10 or more glasses per day.

Finally, whatever your diet, if you do not have at least one soft bowel movement per day, add bulk to your diet. Oat bran is perhaps the tastiest. It can be taken in pill form or eaten as a cereal. If you don't like bran, consider psyllium seed husks, but beware of those brands with 50% sugar! I think I've said enough about alcohol. It's not good for you, but if you do drink, never more than two "drinks" per day!

For caffeinated coffee and tea, try to restrict yourself to two cups per day and none after 4:00 p.m.

Physical Exercise as a Stress Reducer

No single factor influences health and well-being as significantly as does physical activity. Our bodies and minds need activity. Physical activity is as beneficial as smoking is harmful. Physical exercise improves mood, by increasing beta endorphins, the "feel-good" chemicals. The question is not whether to exercise but how and how much. From a Health-Wise point of view, only 23% of Missourians get some exercise. Nationally it may be 25%. This is a great improvement over the 9% reported by Hans Kraus 20 years ago![4]

Posture

Alexander has emphasized the importance of posture.[5] In fact, he and his fellow practitioners believed that many symptoms could be treated with proper posture. Most people slouch, increasingly as the years pass, and have remarkable asymmetries in posture. At least 25% of high school students examined by me for athletic participation have mild to moderate scoliosis, a lateral curvature of the spine. Any deviation of posture from the ideal puts a strain on the entire spine, which has to compensate in order for your head/eyes to be relatively straight in viewing the world. Our inner balancing mechanism demands a certain position of the head in order to avoid feelings of dizziness or unsteadiness. Posture is correlated positively with efficient functioning of the heart and lungs and oxygenation of the tissues.

In more than 8,000 patients seen for problems of chronic pain, virtually all have some asymmetry of posture. That asymmetry contributes to aches, pains, incoordination, weakness, and decreased overall vitality and function. Muscle spasm and strained joints are inevitable consequences.

The first principle of physical fitness then is posture. Alexander therapy, physical therapy, and fitness specialists are your best sources for guidance in posture improvement. Most physicians know little about posture. Most chiropractors "adjust" spinal asymmetry, but do not teach postural alignment.

The ideal posture is almost the military one, without straining the body. Back of head, shoulders, buttocks, calves, and heels should be in an approximate straight line with about a hand's thickness of space behind the knees, low back, and neck. The spine itself should be very straight and symmetrical when viewed from behind, from neck to sacrum, with certain normal differences in the curvature between males and females. Start your Health-Wise exercise program by emphasizing excellent posture.

Strength

General physical energy is a primary manifestation of strength. Beyond that, your general state of energy is related to the strength and tone of various muscles, both internal and external. For a person not involved in heavy physical labor, muscle strength is dependent upon genetic constitution, childhood athletics, and general adult activity. If you are not involved in vigorous sports or "manual" labor, you may not need much specific strength-building exercise.

Most "health clubs" emphasize body building equipment, the modern adaptation of the Charles Atlas consciousness 50 years ago. Although gentle body building is certainly fine and may provide a sense of well-being as well as improved body esthetics, body building through weight resistance training is not nearly as valuable as postural, flexibility, or aerobic exercise. Many teenage weight lifters become flabby in adulthood and increase their risk of heart disease. If you have the time and desire to build muscle mass, do so by integrating muscle strengthening with a conditioning program that integrates attention to posture, flexibility, balance, coordination, and overall toning. On the other hand, if you are going to engage in sports or heavy labor, develop the strength and endurance necessary to avoid injury from tension and strain.

Flexibility

From a feel-good point of view, flexibility exercise is quite as mentally pleasing as aerobic exercise. You can "get by" with 10 to 15 minutes of good flexibility exercise per day. However, after age 50, I believe a half hour or more a day is essential for optimal flexibility. Your program needs to stretch gently each muscle, joint, and tendon through a full range of motion. Many calisthenic and yogic exercise programs are available.

Be sure your instructor is well qualified and makes sense to you. I particularly favor "The Five Rites of Rejuvenation," a special group of exercises republished as *The Eye of Revelation* by Peter Kelder.[6] These can be done in 10 to 15 minutes per day.

Iyengar yoga is also a marvelous technique for optimal flexibility and well-being. I suggest at least a dozen lessons from an Iyengar instructor if you wish to take up this sport. Check the magazine *Yoga*, which is available in many health food stores.

Tai Chi is also a great technique for improving coordination. It requires a longer period of instruction and practice, but is a true meditative art form as well as a very effective body-mind exercise.

Conditioning

Fitness is generally considered to be related to cardiopulmonary endurance or reserves. Actually, it was the wonderful cardiologist Paul Dudley White, President Eisenhower's physician, who introduced Americans to the cardiac benefits of bicycling as exercise. Unfortunately, bicycling has not yet caught on, probably because of the scarcity of urban bikeways in most cities in the United States. Dr. Kenneth Cooper has probably done more to get people involved in the positive benefits in increasing awareness of aerobic activity. Aerobic exercise increases heart rate and strength, lung capacity, and oxygenation. Essentially, any exercise which increases heart rate provides conditioning. (Please note that typically aerobic exercise does not provide adequate flexibility.)

Cooper and his colleagues have presented compelling evidence for the health benefits of physical exercise.[7] Heart disease, high blood pressure, asthma, depression, allergies, and even cancer are all prevented and improved by adequate exercise. Cooper's numerous books are excellent resources. Here are some favorite exercises of mine:

Walking—Walking is one of the safest aerobic exercises. Virtually everyone walks some, and even patients with severe heart disease can walk and increase walking. Dr. George Sheehan, America's running cardiologist, has assured me that you do not need to do a cardiac stress test to take up walking. Remember that a treadmill stress test does carry a slight risk and is a major stress. Although I've had three in the last 14 years, partly for my intellectual curiosity, I have exercised throughout life and am pleased that last year I was still in "olympic fitness." Actually at my age, and in any condition, you can take up walking.

Starting: Wear comfortable, soft-soled shoes, and loose-fitting clothing. How far do you walk, for how long? Observe your routines. Can you walk five minutes without being winded or having discomfort? At this point you may want to spend five minutes before walking doing some gentle limbering of your legs, hips, neck, and shoulders. This will increase your walking comfort.

Start at whatever time is comfortable. Add one minute each day, six days a week. If you experience any added discomfort, stay at that level until you can do it comfortably.

Your Goal: 60 minutes at whatever pace is comfortable. Once you're at 60 minutes, check your distance.

Your Next Goal: Four miles in 60 minutes or a little less. Take at least as long as it took you to get to 60 minutes to reach this speed of walking. Never exceed comfort level. If it is more convenient, you may split your daily walking into two or three equal segments. Take three to six months to reach your goal.

Your Final Walking Goal: Five days of four miles in 60 minutes.

On the sixth day you can do two miles in 30 minutes. On the seventh day rest.

Running on Your Back—Several years ago I created this exercise for those who have back, neck, knee, or hip pain aggravated by walking. It takes virtually all strain off those body areas because of lack of weight bearing.

Starting: Lie on your back, on a firm mattress, exercise pad, or carpet, wear two pairs of socks—old heavy athletic socks are fine. If lying on a carpet, get yourself a carpet remnant for your feet. Now bend one knee, leaving your heel on the floor. As you then straighten that leg, bend the other knee, alternating the two sides just as if you were walking. Once you have a rhythm going, start bending your arms at the elbows alternatively.

Your elbows and feet never leave the surface on which you are lying. This takes all the strain (weight bearing) off the joints. If your back is not comfortable, place a rolled towel beneath the small of your back.

Continue the arm and leg exercise until you feel any fatigue or windedness. Unless you are already in good shape, do not exceed 5 minutes the first day.

Each day add one minute and build to 60 minutes. Gradually increase the speed so that you are moving as rapidly as possible.

This exercise should give you an increase of heart rate (pulse) equal to walking. At optimal speed, heart rate will increase 40 to 50% over your resting baseline.

Goal: Sixty minutes five days a week plus 30 minutes on the sixth day. Play good music while you do this exercise.

Note: Any exercise you can do in natural light (without glasses) gives you a health bonus.

Jogging on a Trampoline—Mini-trampolines can sometimes be more comfortable than walking. Get one in which the mat is attached with a bungie cord for the most pleasant jogging. Always wear good jogging shoes (an athletic shoe store can help).

Starting: Stand on your mini-trampoline first and begin to move your legs and walk in place. Gradually pick up the pace until you are jogging at a comfortable rate. Do not exceed two or three minutes the first day. Each day add one minute and build to 30 minutes, six days a week. Once you are at 30 minutes, gradually increase speed.

Goals: At 120 steps/minute, 40 minutes a day, six days a week.

At 180 steps/minute, 30 minutes a day, six days a week.

At 240 steps/minute, 20 minutes a day, six days a week.

Increase the benefit and fun by getting a pair of Heavy Hands®. Use them gently, and gradually increase weight to a maximum of 10 pounds in each hand. Move your arms in whatever fashion you like. Play good music while you are exercising.

Stationary Bicycle—Use an Aerodyne-type bicycle. Adjust the seat height so that you can sit upright and have your leg still bent 10-15° when the pedal is down. Start pedaling at a pace that is comfortable, and continue a maximum of five minutes.

Each day add one minute and build to 30 minutes, six days a week. Once you are at 30 minutes, gradually increase speed.

Goal: Thirty minutes a day, six days a week, at 35 miles per hour. Do not rush. Take two to six months to reach your goal.

Jogging—Jogging is great exercise and builds beta endorphins better than many other exercises. However, do not take up jogging until you can walk four miles in 59 minutes comfortably.

Starting: Wear good jogging shoes and loose, comfortable clothes. Jog at first on a smooth surface. An athletic track at schools or colleges is ideal.

Start with whatever pace is comfortable and jog slowly until you feel the least bit winded. Then stop. Each day add one minute and build to 30 minutes.

Once you are at 30 minutes, gradually increase speed until you are running two and a half miles in 30 minutes six days a week.

Stay at that pace at least several months. Do not go beyond three miles in 30 minutes. The incidence of injuries increases with faster speeds.

Racquetball—Racquetball is a fantastic sport. Six hours of racquetball equals six hours of brisk walking. Do not take up racquetball or any other more vigorous sport until you can jog two and a half miles in 30 minutes and are limber.

Horseback Riding—No exercise is better for the back. It provides a natural "adjustment" of the spine.

Do not take up riding until you are very limber and in good condition, such as walking six hours per week. Get a competent instructor to start.

Two hours of "average" horseback riding (50% walk, 25% trot, 25% or less canter) is equal to one hour of brisk walking.

Remember: "Halitosis is better than no breath at all." All exercise is good. Create a program that suits you by experimenting. Any is better than none. Nothing can do as much for your health and well-being as adequate physical exercise. Develop a Health-Wise exercise attitude.

Notes—Chapter 9

1. Watson, George, *Nutrition and Your Mind* (New York: Harper & Row Publishers, 1972).

2. Barnes, Broda, "Arteriosclerosis in 10,000 Autopsies and the Possible Role of Dietary Protein," *Federal Proceedings* 19:1 (March 1960).

3. *Statistical Abstract of the U.S.*, 111th Edition (Washington: U.S. Bureau of Census, 1991).

4. Kraus, H., Clinical Treatment of Back and Neck Pain. (New York: McGraw-Hill, 1970).

5 Pevsner, Daniel, "Horsemanship and the Alexander Experience" (lecture in London, England, 1980).

6. Kelder, Peter, *The Eye of Revelation* (Garberville, CA: Borderland Sciences Research Foundation, Inc., 1989).

7. Blair, S.N., H. W. Kohl, R. S. Paffenbarger, D. G. Clark, K. H. Cooper, and L. W. Gibbons,"Physical Fitness and All-Cause Mortality: A Prospective Study of Healthy Men and Women," *JAMA* 262:17 (November 3, 1989): 2395–2401.

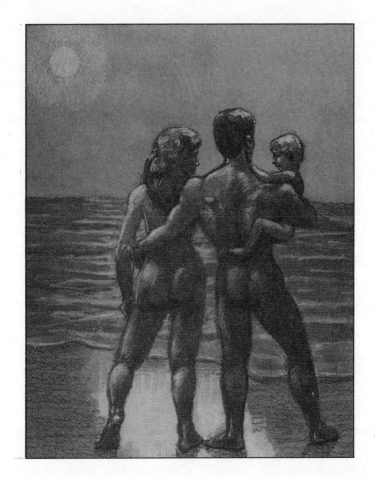

10

Reuniting Body, Mind, and Emotions with Spirit

Of the good in you I can speak, but not of the evil. For what is evil but good tortured by its own hunger and thirst?

The crisis in disease care is a triple one of cost, quality, and control. An epic struggle is entering the final phase. Perhaps it began in the last century with the establishment of the American Medical Association.

Phase two was clearly won by the AMA with the Flexner Report; that report led to closure of half of all hospitals and medical schools. To a large extent, it wiped out most competition: homeopathy, acupuncture, naturopathy. Chiropractic and osteopathy survived, although tremendously wounded; other specialties have suffered near-mortal blows to the detriment of all people who could benefit from their continuations to health care.

Despite the fact that chiropractors have survived tremendous opposition by organized medicine for the past hundred years, they treat almost as many patients as do physicians. And "side effects" are rare. Chiropractors, like all "alternative" practitioners, are notoriouly and erratically reimbursed by the Third Party. They help many more patients with back pain than do physicians. Why should they not be fairly reimbursed? But then what's fair in the Third Party politics?

Osteopathy and chiropractic have gradually recovered and now are being decimated along with allopathy by the Third Party forces, something like the Bolshevik Revolution leading to the dominance of Leninist/Stalinist communism for 74 years. The leaders of the Third Party revolution emerged in the 1920s. Instead of red, they chose blue as their color. Instead of a sickle and hammer, they chose a cross. The Third Party revolution has been relatively more like that promised by Karl Marx—not winning by warfare but by political maneuvering and subterfuge.

With the assistance of the United States presidency, mainly Harry S. Truman and Lyndon B. Johnson, and the U.S. Congress, the third script was clearly complete. The Disease Insurance industry revolution was triumphant. Hospitals quickly capitulated and became eager converts. Together they created *ILL-egalization*, with the rapid infiltration of lawyers into all phases of the revolution to intimidate patients, health care professionals, and any concerned citizens or groups who questioned the revolution's goals. In claiming this power, however, the Third Party system, now an interwoven, semi-integrated den of disease insurance-government-lawyers, and hospitals set the stage for the final phase, the economic and social destruction of the best medical system in the history of the world.

It is true that there are abuses; perhaps 15% of physicians are drug addicts or crooks. It is true that alternatives have been more restricted than in any other country in the world and that new drugs face a greater battle/cost to become "approved" by the czar of the FDA; and it is true that physicians are remarkably resistant to the introduction of new approaches, except drugs and surgery! It is true that despite medicine's public devotion to the scientific double-blind study, proof is lacking for 85% of all currently accepted treatments. It is true that simple approaches such as administration of magnesium after a heart attack could save 70% more lives, but this approach doesn't have the $100-million promotion of a new drug. It is true that in chronic illness drugs and surgery may do more harm than good. It is true that in all this debacle, the patient is the victim, and the Health-Wise the only possible victors.

It is also true that for acute illness, which formerly was the major cause of death and illness, a majority of advances were developed in this country by this same dedicated allopathic system. If allopathy had been allowed to continue, undoubtedly, sooner or later, it would have turned its attention to chronic illness. The emergence of psychoneuroimmunology provides the crown jewel of scientific medicine. Long before psychoneuroimmunology can effect its change on allopathy, however, the Third Party will have destroyed incentive and forced its bureaucratic mediocrity upon the medical profession and disease care.

As a country, it is unlikely that we will develop a system of health care in this century. Most Disease Insurance companies will go belly-up and/or merge into greater Goliaths; the government will then try to institute a nationalized system far more expensive and less effective; and if the country survives bankruptcy by this insanity, eventually common sense will emerge out of chaos. A golden age of health care is possible. The Health-Wise have the potential to begin now. Common sense dictates that somewhere down the road healthy habits will finally interest the government, or we will go bankrupt as a nation. First, however, the Disease Insurance industry will play out its sordid script, hurting, even devastating, a lot of innocent people in the process.

Do not waste your time or energy attempting to convert an insurance company, PPO, HMO, or the government. They are hopelessly as determined as the current hardliners of communism. They can be overcome only by a groundswell of grass-roots pressure. You can fight for a rapid reduction in the number of admissions to medical schools and be ready with creative, profitable uses for bankrupt hospitals. You can support the concept of health care by nonphysicians. Review chapter 1 for more solutions to the crisis.

If the estimated 25% of Americans who are Health-Wise would unite, they could, over a period of five years, force the end of phase four and emerge in control of the situation. The battle would not be peaceful. There are far too many bureaucrats supporting the un-Health-Wise who do not have the will to succeed on their own; there are far too many youngsters, some now adults, who have been retarded by the dissolution of the family. There are far too many who do not understand that the golden goose cannot support the two-thirds who have come to expect a right to disease care, food, and housing without the responsibility of hard work and the personal sacrifice of self-care.

On the other hand, the Health-Wise are willing to take optimal responsibility for themselves and their families. They—you—can make a difference. Individually, you can follow the essential tenets of health:

- No smoking or use of tobacco.
- No or very modest drinking of alcohol.
- No use of narcotics or marijuana.
- No prolonged use of tranquilizers.
- Maintenance of weight within 10% of their ideal.
- Adequate physical exercise.
- Healthy nutrition.
- Seven to eight hours of sleep per night (average).
- A positive mental attitude with planned daily stress reduction.
- A belief in a higher spiritual reality.

You can examine the roots of your own insecurities, educate yourself about healthy living, and nurture yourself with an optimal healthy lifestyle of stress reduction and regular Biogenics®.[1]

You can cut your Disease Insurance costs by 60 to 75% by taking a $5,000 deductible policy and saving the difference. The savings are crucial just in case of an emergency.

You could unite and develop the first real health insurance company, offering disease prevention/health education/stress reduction/wellness programs to supplement the $5,000 deductible plan, with double or triple premiums for the Disease-Wise until they convert.

Your first responsibility is to yourself to preserve your health, to be a role model for family and friends. Only then can you afford to become a crusader for others. A Health-Wise crusader eventually will rise up, bolstered by the growing energies of the Health-Wise, beyond individual health and establish the Foundation for Health. Will s/he emerge before the Third Party destroys itself and the medical profession?

While awaiting this next leap in the Health-Wise crusade, however, health can be yours. May your wisdom empower you to take responsibility to do good to yourself—love yourself enough to continue a Health-Wise life.

Ultimately the way to health is to understand and live the primordial connection of body with mind, emotions, and spirit. Jan Smuts enumerated these principles in the book *Holism and Evolution*.[2] An elegant discourse on the interrelations of the increasingly complex universe, his book laid the foundations for the holistic health movement. Numerous lay organizations—the Holistic Dental Association, American Holistic Medical Association, American Holistic Nurse's Association, and Holistic Veterinary Association—have attracted dedicated visionaries who have a broad vision of a New Age in America. Interestingly, Sir William Osler, the father of American medicine, talked about the New Age one hundred years ago![3] He believed that drugs would not be needed if Americans adopted wise health habits.

The "Establishment" has so far ignored, cursed, or rejected the concepts of holism. Intuitively, however, every Health-Wise person knows that every individual is part of the whole and that every individual is influenced by all others, not only by individuals but by organizations, bureaucracies, other nations, pollution, war, poverty, and every facet of the earth itself.

Ninety percent of people in every society believe in life after death (soul), God, and the golden rule. The very concept of soul is foreign to the Third Party, but integral to the Health-Wise. If we accept the validity of the soul, then we have to accept the reality of an energy not yet "discovered" by science. That energy is consistently interrelated. Interestingly, the obvious connection is through the sun. Life as we experience and know it is totally dependent upon the sun—for heat an7d for light, the form of energy converted by plants into life.

The miracle of life involves the conversion of some basic atoms of the universe, carbon, nitrogen, hydrogen, oxygen, calcium, and magnesium, along with many "trace" elements, into plant "energy." To date, science has not uncovered the secret of converting inert materials into living matter. Undoubtedly, that secret involves some aspect of universal energy related to God and soul.

In one sense, every atom is "alive" with the energy of electrons moving at incredible speeds in their microcosm. In some mysterious, elegant fashion the energy of these atoms and their electrons is transformed by plants into a different behavior, one which begins to be both stronger and weaker than the dormant atomic energy. Undoubtedly, this process involves an atomic conversion more powerful, and more efficient, than the "nuclear" energy of bombs.

Ultimately, all animal and human life is dependent upon plants for their its existence, and plants are dependent upon the sun. Weather patterns that determine rainfall and temperature conditions are dependent upon the sun, moon, and planets for their variations and remarkable consistency.

An even more mysterious energy which "controls" our solar system and its relation with the rest of our vast universe is likely. This unifying cosmic energy unites all atoms with one another in some interpenetrating fashion.

The physical body is one manifestation of the ever more complex organization of universal energy. The mind, the most mysterious aspect of life, and our hands and our speech are the major features which distinguish us from other forms of life. Emotions represent the reactions of our body to our belief systems, our attitudes towards every aspect of existence. Emotions are physical feelings accompanying biochemical changes induced by fear, anger, guilt, anxiety, depression, or joy.

Ultimately, as Viktor Frankl emphasized in *Man's Search for Meaning*, despots can take away everything, including life, except for our choice of attitude towards circumstances.[4] The will to choose appears to be the basic connection of human beings to their inner ideals at a soul level. Even the "Third Party" is composed of individuals who have a choice. Intuition tells us that at a soul level we are all united in our basic belief in the golden rule. It is not an easy rule; it is simple. Treat other people well or they will get even with you. Common sense and experience demonstrate this principle daily. Beyond common sense there is an ultimate unifying need, that of an insatiable desire to nurture and to be nurtured.

The Health-Wise seek to express this desire to do good in their thoughts and actions. They are united in an attitude of love. The expression of that love will eventually provide the energy to transform the immature behavior of the Third Party into a nurturing one.

Many years ago Martha Guidici, a wonderful Unity minister, assisted me in understanding that "evil" is just immaturity. Three hundred years ago, Saddam Hussein would have been a world hero because of his abuse of power. Despite the vigor with which I have criticized the Third Party, I know that each person making up the Third Party has an Inner Being that is magnificent, wise, and loving. Unfortunately, the personality is not always guided by that inner wisdom.

Discernment says that what I have called evil is really immaturity, living a non-golden rule existence. When the Third Party awakens its golden rule consciousness, a Golden Age will emerge. Until that time, the Health-Wise can use their desire to do good by uniting their energy to create optimal health for themselves and their families. Their example will be of transcendent value to all.

Notes—Chapter 10

1. Shealy, C. Norman, *90 Days to Self-Health* (New York: Dial Press, 1977).

2. Smuts, Jan C., *Holism and Evolution* (New York: The MacMillan Company, 1926).

3. Osler, Sir William, *Aequanimitas*, 3rd Edition (Philadelphia: The Blakiston Company, 1943).

4. Frankl, Viktor E., *Man's Search for Meaning* (New York: Washington Square Books, 1985).

Epilogue

A Case in Point

On February 17, 1988, our clinic was certified by the appropriate federal agencies to become a Comprehensive Outpatient Rehabilitation Facility, or CORF. This is a program mandated by Congress to provide rehabilitation services for the elderly and those on Medicare. The intermediary to whom we were assigned was Blue Cross/Blue Shield of St. Louis.

From the beginning of our certification, we were virtually totally unable to have any cooperation or even to have a decent dialogue with Blue Cross/Blue Shield. They would not tell us what was required for billing or documenting, and they initially sent us the wrong forms for billing. Finally, through intense pressure on our part, over nine months after we have been certified and had been required to bill only through this program and accept assignment for such treatment, we had a preliminary meeting with Blue Cross/Blue Shield. They then came to visit us in our clinic, and on December 19, ten months later, we finally received some guidelines in which they were already deciding that they would deny most of the therapy that we carried out at the Institute. Eventually they actually denied the vast majority of all charges. Within six months of learning that it was quite obvious that we would not be able to provide the services without losing the vast majority of the money and essentially going bankrupt if we had a lot of Medicare patients, we dropped out as a CORF provider. Not only had they denied our charges, but when we applied for administrative and cost overhead, Blue Cross/Blue

Shield, in an extremely sloppy and inadequate audit, and what they themselves even admitted was "our limited audit," denied all administrative overhead. They decided it hadn't cost us anything to do the program!

We appealed both these decisions. Finally in November 1992 a hearing was held before a federal Medicare judge. The expert witness at this hearing was a rheumatologist. She testified that all of our services were necessary and essential for the patients' welfare, and were the standard of care at pain clinics throughout the country. Subsequently the Medicare judge decided totally in our favor that all of our charges were legitimate and that Medicare should fully reimburse us.

Meanwhile, the appeal for the administrative overhead and costs had to go through separate channels through the HCFA office itself. Less than two weeks prior to the hearing that was to be held in Washington, DC, and after extensive work on our part and legal expense, we received a call from an accountant of Blue Cross/Blue Shield of Chicago who said that the case had been turned over to him, and he thought that based upon our position paper it was obvious that we had a good negotiating position and that he thought we should cancel the hearing in Washington and would be able to settle this equitably out of court.

An interesting sideline is that Blue Cross/Blue Shield of St. Louis in early 1992 withdrew from being a Medicare provider because they said that their administrative overhead was not being adequately reimbursed! It couldn't have happened to a nicer group.

Annotated Bibliography

Following is a brief review of some sources worth reading. I have quoted highlights to assist you in deciding whether to read the originals. In addition, I have searched hundreds of other articles and books not quoted. The self-help, self-health literature is extensive.

Abraham, Laurie. "Regulation Opponents Told They Should Quit Medicine." *American Medical News* (8/15 July 1988): 21.

> According to Uwe Reinhardt, Ph.D., "You're entering the market for a commodity that is widely perceived as a social good ... If you don't want government interference, get out of medicine."

Abraham, Laurie. "Transplants Available—For Young, White, Wealthy Men." *American Medical News* (7 January 1991): 24.

> "Medicare covers dialysis and transplant surgery, but provides only limited coverage of immunosuppressive drugs needed to prevent rejection."

> Interestingly, one-third of the patients waiting for transplants nationwide are black, with only 10% of donors being black.

"ACPM Salary Survey Indicates Preventive Medicine Physicians Earn Less." *ACPM News* (July/August 1991): 1, 8.

> "The median income for preventive medicine physicians of $84,600" is definitely below the 1989 median income for all physicians, which was $125,000. The average physician now earns approximately the same as a U.S. Congressperson, but only 20% of the average income of a major league baseball player.

Airing, Charles. "A Random Patient Consulting a Physician at Random." *JAMA* 229:7 (12 August 1974): 785–6.

This article states that Lawrence J. Henderson, opined that "somewhere between 1910 and 1912 in this country, a random patient with a random disease, consulting a doctor chosen at random had, for the first time in the history of mankind, a better than fifty-fifty chance of profiting from the encounter."

Altman, Stuart H., and Robert Blendon. "Report of the Symposium." In Stuart H. Altman and Robert Blendon (eds.). *Medical Technology: The Culprit Behind Health Care Costs* (proceedings of the 1977 Sun Valley Forum on National Health). Washington: United States Department of Health, Education, and Welfare; U.S. Government Printing Office, 297, 302.

A definition of third parties: "The government and insurance companies."

"Medical technology per se is not the culprit behind rising costs in health care."

"America's Doctors." *U.S. News & World Report* (17 October 1977): 50–8.

The author says, "Today only one-seventh of the country's physicians are in primary care—general practice—although 90% of the problems that send patients to doctors do not require any specialty training."

The article quotes Dr. William J. Barclay, at that time editor of the *JAMA*, who states, "Practicing medicine is no longer any fun."

He stated that medicine was shifting toward more preventive measures and self-care programs, but in the next 16 years I certainly haven't seen that.

Anderson, Kevin. "Health Care Costs More, Serves Fewer." *USA Today* (11 March 1991): 1B–2B.

Medical expenses were $2,700 per American in 1990.

The article quotes one woman who pays 44% of her take-home pay for family insurance coverage. Although her daughter's leukemia has been dormant for 15 years, no insurance company will cover them.

Total medical spending in 1965 was $41.6 billion. By 1980 it was a bit more than $200 billion. By 1990 it was $600 billion. It is estimated that by 1995 it will be about $950 billion and that by the year 2000 it will be $1.5 trillion.

Medical expenses per person in 1965 were $204, and as we already said, were $2,700 in 1990. In 1965, medical expenses were 5.9% of the gross national product, and in 1990 they were 15% of the gross national product.

There are 37 million people in the United States without any medical insurance; 49% are working adults, 33% are dependent children, and 18% are nonworking adults.

Anderson, Kevin. "Reform Plans Focus on Access, Cost of Care." *USA Today* (11 March 1991): 3B.

In 1949, 47% of the population recommended a government financed medical insurance. In 1965, when Medicare came in, it was 63%. It dropped to 50% in 1980, but 65% now favor it in 1989. Only 22%, however, stated that they would support an increase of more than $200 in taxes to provide such a system.

Anderson, Kevin. "Technology Fuels Health-Care Inflation." *USA Today* (11 March 1991): 3B.

According to this article, payrolls of hospitals take up more than 70% of the average budget. Generally it's believed that technology and the work force are the major costs involved.

Anderson, Kevin. "Why Health-Care Costs are Tough to Cure." *USA Today* (11 March 1991): 3B.

Seventy-five per cent of adults say they have a doctor they consider to be their family's physician. Fifty-three per cent rate the quality of their doctor's care as excellent, and 39% as good.

One person in four was hospitalized in the past year. Forty-seven per cent rated their hospital care as excellent, and 35% as good. As far as the so-called health care system, only 6% considered it excellent, 32% good.

Anderson, Kevin. "Group Sheds Light on Medical Pariahs." *USA Today* (20 June 1991).

They report that citizen action has found an inside "medical underwriting guide" of an "unnamed major health insurer."

They estimate that 81 million Americans, that is 37% of the population under age 65, have one or more of the conditions that the guide will flag as risky and that all 81 million of those individuals are at risk of losing health insurance. Basically, it would exclude coverage for costs associated with 78 conditions in new applicants ranging from acne through angina, bone spurs, bunions, discs, headaches, etc. In other words, if you have had any illness, they would exclude you from new coverage; would raise rates 50% to 140% for people who develop some 49 different illnesses; and deny all coverage for applicants with a wide variety of other illnesses. In other words, the medical insurance industry is on the verge of taking your money but covering nothing!

"Bad Faith: Insurance Companies Claim-Review Process Operated in Conscious Disregard of Insured's Rights." *Litigation and Insurance Dispatch* (November 1989). From Reed, Elliott, Creech & Roth, a professional corporation of lawyers in San Jose, California.

"An insured submitted several claims to Blue Cross resulting from her son's medically authorized stays in a psychiatric institution. Blue Cross denied the majority of the claims after an 'investigation.' After a trial, a jury awarded the insured $150,000 in compensatory damages and $700,000 in punitive damages for Blue Cross's breech of its covenant of good faith and fair dealing. Blue Cross appealed, arguing that the verdict was unsupported by the evidence. The Court of Appeal affirmed the judgment and held that there was ample evidence to support the verdict because it was shown that Blue Cross conducted a cursory review of the medical records, used a standard of medical necessity at variance with community standards, and issued uninformative denial letters to the treating physicians. The appellate court held that the duty of good faith implies consistency with the justified expectations of the insured and that Blue Cross's restricted definitions of medical necessity, which was at variance with community medical standards, frustrated the justified expectations of the insured. Hughes v. Blue Cross of Northern California (November 1989, First District) 89 C.D.O.S. 8338."

Beals, Rodney, K., and Norman Hickman. "Industrial Injuries of the Back and Extremities." *The Journal of Bone and Joint Surgery* 54A:8 (December 1972): 1593–1611.

At that time they stated that millions of Americans are injured in industrial accidents, and 1.2 million Americans sustained back injuries annually. Sixty-five per cent of those had some permanent disability, and at that time approximately 2.5 million Americans had permanent impairment of the back as a result of injury.

They found that physical and psychological disability play an important role in a return to work in both extremity injured and back-
injured individuals.

"Injured workers were significantly more anxious, depressed, and
preoccupied with physical and emotional symptoms than the
employed workman."

Only 39% of back-operated workers' compensation injured individuals returned to work within two years.

Berk, Aviva A., and Thomas C. Chalmers. "Cost and Efficacy of the Sub-
stitution of Ambulatory for Inpatient Care." *New England Journal of
Medicine* 304:7 (12 February 1981): 393–7.

The authors studied 134 papers and found that only four provided
enough data on cost and efficiency to allow for statistically valid conclusions. "Two of these four demonstrated that potential savings
would be accompanied by a slightly poorer clinical outcome; two
showed ambulatory care to be as effective as inpatient care and less
costly."

Blair, Steven N., et. al. "Physical Fitness and Incidence of Hypertension in
Healthy Normotensive Men and Women." *JAMA* 252:4 (27 July
1984): 487–90.

Physical fitness was measured by maximal treadmill testing in 4,820
men and 1,219 women age 20–65. Individuals with a low level of
physical fitness (72% of the group) had a relative risk of 1.52 for the
development of hypertension when compared to a very fit person.

Blendon, Robert J., and Thomas W. Molony. "Perspectives on the Grow-
ing Debate Over the Cost of Medical Technologies." In Stuart H. Alt-
man and Robert Blendon (eds.). *Medical Technology: The Culprit Behind
Health Care Costs* (proceedings of the 1977 Sun Valley Forum on
National Health). Washington: United States Department of Health,
Education, and Welfare; U.S. Government Printing Office, 11–2.

"The Great Society legislation included two government programs,
one designed to offset medical care for the aging, the other for the
poor. The enactment of these two programs sparked the beginning of
the large-scale growth of American public insurance and the dramatic increase in federal budgetary contributions to the health sector."

They quote that $39 billion was spent on medical care in 1965, but by

1972 health medical expenditures increased to almost $83.5 billion. Inflation accounted for $22.25 billion.

Please note that between 1950 and 1970 physician fees increased approximately 200% while hospital daily service charges increased approximately 500%. It is worth noting that population increased 9.9% during that same time, or from 1965 to 1972 all items increased an average of 33%, food increased 31%, transportion 25%, medical care 48%, and hospital charges for a semi-private room 129%.

Bowen, Wanda. "Medicine in the Good Old Days." *Private Practice* 20:5 (May 1988): 44.

"Years ago, you left your office with happiness because you had helped someone. Now you leave with anger and sadness because you can't practice like years ago."

That author goes on to say, "We're seeing less compassion and more greed. The government and insurance companies tell doctors how and when they can care for patients and how long patients can stay in the hospital."

Brostoff, Steven. "U.S. Spends $604 Billion on Health Care in '89." *National Underwriter* (7 January 1991): 3.

Nineteen per cent went to physician services, 39% to hospital care, 8% to nursing home care. Seventeen per cent of the money came from Medicare, 10% from Medicaid, 15% from other government programs. Private so-called health insurance covered 33%, 21% was considered "out of pocket", and from somewhere else in the private sector came another 4%.

Bruce, Thomas. "Attending to the Business of Health Care." In *Stemming the Rising Costs of Medical Care: Answers and Antidotes.* Battlecreek, MI: W. K. Kellogg Foundation, 1988.

"The hospital/health care business is among the three largest industries in the country, whether measured by employment or dollars spent" (p. 51).

To be quite honest, I didn't learn much from reading this entire book, despite the aims in the title.

Burchfield, Susan R., et. al. "Personality Differences Between Sick and Rarely Sick Individuals." *Social Science Medicine* 15B, 145–8.

"Satisfaction appeared to be linearly related to health status: as satisfaction decreased, frequency of illness increased."

Interestingly, "rarely sick people seldom worried or felt uptight, while sick individuals reported feeling chronically uptight and worried."

Burkitt, Denis. "Are our Commonest Diseases Preventable?" *The Pharos* (Winter 1991): 19–21.

"It has been estimated that Western man has made more change in his life-style, and in his eating habits in particular, in the last 200-300 years than in the previous 20,000 years."

He implicates the dietary changes as being major etiological factors in disease. He ends up by stating, "We're making great progress, but we're headed in the wrong direction."

Burnum, John F. "The Malaise in Internal Medicine." *Archives of Internal Medicine* 137 (February 1977).

Actually this frustration and chaos evident in physician-Third Party relations is well into its second decade. And the concept of "rationing" as raised by Aaron and Schwartz has been around also since at least 1977.

Dr. Burnum states, "Internists today are discomforted by uncertainty of identity, governmental interference with practice, total responsibility for patients' health, and by waning of faith in science."

Burnum emphasizes the problems of increasing governmental control of health care patterns for financing. He states, "We will not be able to provide health care for all at some tolerable cost without controls and rationing of health care resources."

"Can You Afford to Get Sick?" *Newsweek* (30 January 1989): 44–51.

Total medical expenditures were 5.9% of gross national product in 1965 and 11.1% in 1987.

They quote one worker who said, "In my old job I had to call the insurance company every time I made a move. Changing employers was the only way I could survive."

Some other interesting comparisons ... A chest X-ray in 1979, $27.50; in 1989, $59; a cesarean section in 1979, $5,010; in 1989, $10,900.

They quote Joseph Califano, former secretary of HEW, saying, "By the year 2000, the only person in the United States who can afford to get sick will be Donald Trump." That, of course, was before Trump's problems!

Cooper, Barbara S., and Clifton R. Gaus. "Controlling Health Technology." In Stuart H. Altman and Robert Blendon (eds.). *Medical Technology: The Culprit Behind Health Care Costs* (proceedings of the 1977 Sun Valley Forum on National Health). Washington: United States Department of Health, Education, and Welfare; U.S. Government Printing Office, 260.

It was recommended that within the next five years there would be a decrease of at least 10% in the ratio of short-term general hospital beds and "further significant reductions thereafter."

Davis, Jay M. "Food Insurance and Individual Health Accounts." *Western Journal of Medicine* 129 (December 1978): 518–520.

Dr. Davis suggests an "Individual Health Account." The person is to make monthly payments into that, but if the individual does not use the money, it remains his or hers. If an individual goes to a doctor or uses any medical services, the bill is paid with a check on that account. There is a maximum amount of money required in an IHA.

"The failure of private health insurance is evident from the skyrocketing cost of premiums. The failure of federal programs is seen in massive cost overruns and the near bankruptcy of the Social Security System."

The state would pay for those individuals who are not working.

Consistently he says this system would get rid of 25–50% of every "health" dollar that goes for administration.

Davis, Karen, et. al. "Paying for Preventive Care: Moving the Debate Forward." *American Journal of Preventive Medicine* 6:4 (1990).

It's estimated that total lifetime costs for delivering preventive services would be $2,898 for a male and $4,683 for a female, or an average cost per year over an entire lifetime of $34 per male and $55 per female. This includes physician visits, all recommended immunizations, urinalysis, hematocrit, cholesterol tests, glaucoma testing, mammography, and Pap smears in women, etc. Of course it does not include real prevention, which is education and self-regulation training!

Drake, Jinx. "A Current Interest." *Coastlines* (May-June 1976). A reprint by Coastal States Life Insurance Companies.

"'A man was arrested yesterday, charged with attempting to obtain money under false pretenses. He claimed he was promoting a device whereby one person could talk to another several miles away, by means of a small apparatus and some wire. Without doubt this man is a fraud and an unscrupulous trickster and must be taught that the American public is too smart to be the victim of this and similar schemes. Even if this insane idea worked, it would have no practical value other than for circus side shows'. A short time later, in 1876, Alexander Graham Bell took out a patent on the telephone. (Reprint from a newspaper clipping of 1876)."

The author suggests that insurance companies hedge their bets "by designing and selling plans that will promote and program people to live longer and healthier, that inspires the desire to do so."

"On future health insurance policies ... we should design plans that would program and motivate people for health. It can be so constructed as to reward a policyholder for remaining healthy and to penalize him for being sick. Money is one whale of a motivation for being healthy and even to go on living."

"The medicine of the future is preventive medicine."

Dreyfuss, Ira. "Moderate Exercise Boosts Immune System." *News-Leader* (Saturday, 30 March 1991): 4C.

David C. Nieman, associate professor of health, leisure, and exercise science at Appalachian State University in North Carolina cites the following information.

Interestingly, it's moderate exercise, not extremely heavy duty exercise, that is important. For instance, more than 13% of 2,300 runners in the 1987 Los Angeles Marathon came down with a cold or flu within a week afterwards, compared with only 2% of those who trained but didn't compete.

In the two months before the race approximately 40% got sick. Those who trained more than 60 miles a week had twice the risk than those who trained less than 20 miles a week.

He actually advises that "serious athletes" do no more than two intense workouts per week.

Indeed, moderate exercise such as a 45-minute brisk walk five days a week increases immunity, and such individuals have half the cold/flu days of nonwalking colleagues.

"Dr. Weed Sounds Off for POMR." *Medical Group News* 7:7 (July 1974): 1, 4.

Dr. Lawrence L. Weed, professor of medicine at the University of Vermont, states that overutilization "is killing American medicine" through "overdiagnosis, overtreatment, and overmedication." He states that a big reason is overlapping of effort because of poor record keeping.

"Editor Fired: AMA Denies Medical Crisis." *LaCrosse Tribune* (Friday, 7 February 1975): 4.

This article stated that it appeared that Bard Lindeman was suspensed as editor-in-chief of *Today's Health* by the AMA because he wrote about "The Crisis in Medical Care." Basically he was just talking about the prices, talked about in many other places, as far as cost for medical care.

Efaith, Margaret, et. al. "The Cost of Continuing Medical Education for Family Physicians." *JAMA* 242 (3 August 1979): 449–50.

At that time the average family practice physicians spent approximately $5,353 each year for attendance at formal continuing medical education activities. Triple that today.

Enthoven, Alain, and Roger Noll. "Regulatory and Nonregulatory Strategies for Controlling Health Care Costs." In Stuart H. Altman and Robert Blendon (eds.). *Medical Technology: The Culprit Behind Health Care Costs* (proceedings of the 1977 Sun Valley Forum on National Health). Washington: United States Department of Health, Education, and Welfare; U.S. Government Printing Office.

"A study by the National Academy of Sciences found in the Veterans' Administration Hospital "that about half the patients in acute medical beds, one-third of the patients in surgical beds, and over half the patients in psychiatric beds did not require or receive services for the specialized medical facilities that were associated with these types of beds. The Veterans' Administration experience reflects a pervasive problem that government encounters when it tries to provide services directly to citizens."

Evans, Roger. "Health Care Technology and the Inevitability of Resource Allocation and Rationing Decisions, Part II." JAMA 249:16 (22/29 April 1983: 2208–19.

"The resources available to meet the demand for health care are limited.

Farber, Emmanuel. "Chemical Carcinogenesis." *New England Journal of Medicine* 305:23 (3 December 1981): 1379–89.

"About one-third of the cancer in North America and Europe is related to the use of cigarettes or other tobacco products."

"Few Insurers Offer Broad Coverage for Preventive Care." *American Medical News* (14 March 1986): 29.

"Only 6% of the nation's medical insurance companies cover most of the common preventive medicine claims."

Only 26% cover stress management programs, annual physicals, or nutritional education. Only 11% cover smoking cessation programs. Eighty-nine per cent of the insurance companies said that they would "never" cover smoking cessation unless required to do so by law. But 68% cover alcohol abuse treatment, and 66% cover drug abuse programs. Thirty-eight per cent cover weight control programs, and 40% cover monitored exercise plans.

Interestingly, 86% of employees would like somewhat or very much to have preventive medical insurance coverage.

Fielding, Jonathan E. "Smoking: Health Effects and Control, Part I." *New England Journal of Medicine* 313:9 (22 August 1985): 491–8.

"The estimated annual excess mortality from cigarette smoking in the United States exceeds 350,000 more than the total number of American lives lost in World War I, Korea, and Vietnam combined, and almost as many as were lost in World War II."

At least 30% of the 565,000 annual deaths from coronary artery disease, or a total of 170,000 deaths, are attributed to smoking. Also, 30% of the 412,000 annual cancer deaths, or about 125,000 are attributed to smoking, with 80% resulting in carcinoma of the lung. Emphysema and chronic obstructive diseases account for another 62,000 smoking related deaths each year.

"It has been estimated that an average of $5\frac{1}{2}$ minutes of life is lost for each cigarette smoked."

In fact, "the overwhelming cause of male-female longevity differences and the increases in life expectancy between the sexes since 1930 are largely attributable to cigarette smoking."

As of 1985 it was estimated that the direct health medical costs associated with smoking were in excess of $16 billion, with another $37 billion attributed to lost productivity and earnings, or an annual per capita social cost directly attributed to smoking of approximately $200.

"The economic burden on each nonsmoker for providing medical care for smoking induced illness exceeds $100, paid primarily through taxes and health insurance premiums."

Smoking is also responsible for one-quarter of all the mortality caused by fire, and causes close to $500 million in other losses.

Fielding, Jonathan E. "Smoking: Health Effects and Control, Part 2." *New England Journal of Medicine* 313:9, 555–61.

"Smokers uniformly use more employer-sponsored health benefits and are absent more days per year." For instance, the average smoker is absent 5.5 more days per year and has eight more days of disability leave per year.

"Conservative estimates of the excess costs to employers incurred by each smoker are in the range of $300 to $800 per year (1984 dollars)."

"In 1982, consumers spent close to $25 billion on tobacco products, which is equal to 1.2% of all personal disposable income and 6% of the total spent on nondurable goods."

Actually, overall, the total annual contribution of tobacco to the national economy is $2^{1}/_{2}$% of the gross national product. Interestingly, "domestic tobacco exports account for 5% of all U.S. exports."

Fishman, Howard. "Hawaii Medicaid Fraud Unit Guilty of Malicious Prosecution." *The Psychiatric Times* 6:8 (August 1989).

A Hawaii clinical psychologist, Dr. Leonard Licht, was awarded $600,000 in damages because it was felt there was "clear and convincing proof" that the Hawaiian Medicaid organization was "motivated by malice and not by otherwise proper purpose."

"Licht is one of several dozen Medicaid providers, many of them mental health professionals, who were subjected to what has been described in testimony before the Hawaii legislature as a 'reign of terror' conducted by 'goon squads' which regularly use 'gestapo tactics.'"

Fitzgerald, John F., et. al. "The Care of Elderly Patients with Hip Fracture: Changes Since Implementation of the Prospective Payment System." *New England Journal of Medicine* 319:21 (24 November 1988): 1392–7.

The length of hospitalization decreased from 21.9 to 12.6 days. Inpatient physical therapy decreased from 7.6 to 6.3 sessions, and the maximal distance walked before discharge from the hospital fell from 27 to 11 meters, while the proportion of patients discharged from nursing homes rose from 38% to 60%, and those remaining in nursing homes one year after hospitalization rose from 9% to 33%. In-hospital and one year mortality did not change significantly.

"Fruits, Vegetables Might Cut Lung Cancer Risk." *Daily News* (13 November 1986), 5B.

The article reports on a study in which it was found that fruits and vegetables may cut lung cancer rates.

Geyman, John P. "Future Medical Practice in the United States: A Choice of Scenarios." *JAMA* 245:11 (1981), 1140–3.

Interestingly, the author mentions a 1966 study which "painted a bleak scenario for 1990."

That author had predicted that medicine would be practiced on an assembly line, that private practice would no longer exist, and that most physicians would be full-time employees of a medical center complex.

The author says that at that time there were 437,000 physicians in the country, representing a 68% increase since 1960 and a 30% increase since 1970.

He states that it was the general consensus that at least 50% of medical graduates should enter primary care such as family practice, general internal medicine, and general pediatrics.

He talks about health expenditures doubling from 4.5% to 9% of gross national product in the previous 20 years, with expectations to exceed 10% by 1991.

Goodwin, James S., et. al. "Association Between Nutritional Status and Cognitive Functioning in. a Healthy Elderly Population." *JAMA* 249 (1983): 2917–21.

In 260 noninstitutionalized men and women older than 60 years of age with no known physical illnesses and no medication, nutritional status was evaluated. Subjects with low blood levels of vitamin C or B12 scored worse on the Halstead-Reitan Categories Test and the Wechsler Memory Test. Subjects with low levels of riboflavin and folic acid scored worse on the Categories Test. They concluded that "subclinical malnutrition may play a small role in the depression of cognitive function detectable in some elderly individuals, or depressed cognitive function may result in reduced nutrient intake."

Greenfield, Sheldon, et. al. "Efficiency and Cost of Primary Care by Nurses & Physician Assistants." *New England Journal of Medicine* 298 (9 February 1978): 305–9.

In a study of 472 patients with four common acute complaints (respiratory infections, urinary and vaginal infections, headache, and abdominal pain), physician time per patient was reduced by 92% and average visit costs were 20% less.

Gross, Stanley J. "The Myth of Professional Licensing." *American Psychologist* (November 1978): 1009–15.

"Rather, the evidence reveals licensing to be a mystifying arrangement that promises protection of the public, but that actually institutionalizes a lack of accountability to the public. The collusion between the state and the professionals is maintained by myth. Acknowledging the failure of licensing is preparatory to defining the problem of how to protect the public."

"The history of licensing in the health professions centers on the attempts of special interests to impose or to sabotage a monopoly on the practice of healing."

Grumet, Gerald W. "Health Care Rationing Through Inconvenience: The Third Party's Secret Weapon." *New England Journal of Medicine* 321:9 (31 August 1989): 607–11.

"Paradoxically, the savings that ordinarily accrue to an efficiently managed business are reversed in the case of insurance carriers, whose bungling, confusion, and delay impede the outflow of funds. For carriers, inefficiency is profitable."

Because of the increased bureaucracy imposed by the medical insurance industry, it is now estimated that "each visit to a physician's office is estimated to generate ten pieces of paper."

There is a great deal of warring between carriers.

Havighurst, Clark C., and Glenn M. Hackbarth. "Private Cost Containment." *New England Journal of Medicine* 300:23, 1298–1305.

This article argues for a more competitive health medical insurance market.

Health Lawyers News Report 16:6 (May 1988).

The Inspector General's Office of the Department of Health and Human Services concluded that in 1985 the nation's hospitals over-charged Medicare by $2 billion. They found at that time 10.5% of patients were admitted unnecessarily to hospitals.

Healthy People: the Surgeon General's Report on Health Promotion and Disease Prevention. Washington: United States Department of Health, Education, and Welfare, 1979.

"Let's make no mistake about the significance of this document. It represents an emerging consensus among scientists and the health community that the Nation's health tragedy must be dramatically recast to emphasize the prevention of disease" (p.vii).

"You, the individual, can do more for your own health and well-being than any doctor, any hospital, any drug, any exotic medical device" (p. viii).

"Indeed, a wealth of scientific research reveals that the key to whether a person will be healthy or sick, live a long life or die pre-maturely, can be found in several simple personal habits: one's habits with regard to smoking and drinking; one's habits of diet, sleep, and exercise; whether one obeys the speed laws and wears seat belts; and a few other simple measures" (pp. viii-ix).

It is worth emphasizing that in 1977 major cardiovascular diseases accounted for roughly 50% of all deaths, with cancer accounting for just over 20%.

The United States lags behind other industrial nations. Twelve others do better in preventing deaths from cancer; 26 others have a lower death rate from circulatory disease; 11 others do a better job of keeping babies alive in the first year of life; and 14 others have a higher level of life expectancy for men and 6 others have a higher level for women (p. 6).

"Cigarette smoking is the single most important preventable cause of death" (p. 7).

"Alcohol is a factor in more than 10% of all deaths in the United States" (p. 7).

"Within the practical grasp of most Americans are simple measures to enhance the prospects of good health, including:

• elimination of cigarette smoking;

- reduction of alcohol misuse;

- moderate dietary changes to reduce intake of excess calories, fat, salt, and sugar;

- moderate exercise;

- periodic screening for major disorders such as high blood pressure and certain cancers; and

- adherance to speed laws and use of seat belts" (p. 10).

"Disease and disability are not inevitable events to be experienced equally by all" (p. 13).

"Many of today's most pressing health problems are related to excesses—of smoking, drinking, faulty nutrition, overuse of medications, fast driving, and relentless pressure to achieve" (p. 14).

Of the ten leading causes of death, at least seven could be substantially reduced if Americans improved poor diet, smoking, lack of exercise, alcohol abuse, and use of anti-hypertensive medication (p. 14).

"Some 70,000 prescription drugs (with 2,000 individual ingredients) are now on the market, along with 200,000 over-the-counter preparations. Each year 15 to 20 new chemical entities are introduced. In 1977, 1.4 billion prescriptions were filled at a cost of about $8 billion" (p. 115).

"Thirty-five percent of women between ages 45 and 64 with incomes below poverty level and 29% of those with incomes above are considered obese ... The comparable figures for men are five and 13%" (p. 129).

"Cigarette smoking is the principle preventable cause of chronic disease and death in this country" (p. 152).

Helmrich, S.P., et. al. "Physical Activity and Reduced Occurrence of Non-Insulin-Dependent Diabetes Mellitus." *New England Journal of Medicine* 325 (1991): 147–52.

In following some 5,990 male alumni of the University of Pennsylvania from 1962 to 1976, it was found that 202 of the men developed non-insulin-dependent diabetes mellitus during 98,524 "man years." The incidence of diabetes decreased as energy expenditures increased from less than 5 kcal to 3500 kcal per week. Thus an individual who expended 3500 kcal had a 42% less chance of developing diabetes than one who expended less than 500 kcal. And this association is totally independent of diabetes, hypertension, and a family history of diabetes, with the greatest protection coming to those with the greatest risk.

Hofmann, James, et. al. "The Effect of Surgery on Cellular Immunity." *Wisconsin Medical Journal* 72 (December 1973): 249–253.

The bottom line is following both partial gastrectomy and inguinal herniorrhaphy there is significant depression of the immune function with returns to pre-operative level by the fourth day for herniorrhaphy and by the 21st day for the gastrectomy group.

"Hospital Closures Set Record." *Columbia* (MO) *Daily Tribune* (22 March 1989).

For the sixth consecutive year, a record number of community hospitals closed their doors last year, with 81 community hospitals in 28 states shutting down in 1988. Forty-three of those were rural.

Since 1980, 445 community hospitals have closed. In addition, there were 21 noncommunity hospitals closing in 1988, bringing the total number of hospital closures to 102.

Howard, Elliott, J. *Health Risks*. Tucson: The Body Press, 1986.

"Men who are 20% overweight live 20% shorter lives than normal weight men. Women who are 20% overweight live 10% shorter lives than normal weight women" (chap. 11. p. 33).

"Men who have physically active jobs have less coronary artery disease than men with sedentary jobs."

"Brain scans of people who drink alcohol heavily on a daily basis show their brains slowly atrophy."

"Lowering the average in cholesterol level in an experimental group by 10% lowers the group's incidence of coronary disease by 23%."

In obese people (those 30% or more above their ideal weight), sudden cardiac arrest is four times more common than it is in people close to their ideal weight.

"Smoking accounts for 75% of all lung cancer."

"People who smoke have about 20% less oxygen in their blood than nonsmokers!"

"If you smoke and have a high cholesterol level, you are compounding your risk four times."

"Smoking one pack of cigarettes a day triples the risk of a death from coronary heart disease compared to the risk for a nonsmoker."

Hughes, Robert G., et. al. "Are We Mortgaging the Medical Profession?" *New England Journal of Medicine* 325:6 (8 August 1991): 404–7.

In 1989–1990 the median tuition for state residents at public medical schools was $5,810, while as for private medical schools it was $17,794. Resident tuition at public schools has increased 277% since 1960 and in private schools 403% after adjustment for inflation.

Interestingly, in 1960-1961 income from clinical practices of faculty members was only 3% of total revenues that they received. by 1988–1989 that share had risen to 27.4%. And during the same period of time, full-time medical school faculty members increased from 11,224 to 70,300, with the ratio of full-time faculty members to medical students increasing from 0.37 to 1.08.

Actually tuition makes up only 15.4% of expenditures for teaching and training in state schools, 8% in public schools, and 27.2% in private schools.

The average debt for medical school graduates in 1990 was $46,220, an increase of 77% since 1980.

The authors conclude that it might be possible for doctors to meet the health and medical cares of underserved populations in exchange for tuition-free medical education, with the government providing their medical education if they would be willing to spend some time in the public health service.

Hunter, Thomas H. "On Letting Die." *Pharos* (January 1977): 31.

He states, "The consequences of keeping alive unwisely are becoming more and more obvious and will force us to examine our practices squarely and openly."

Hussey, Hugh H. "Too Many Physicians: Sound Alarm!" *JAMA* 245:12 (27 March 1981): 1252.

The Graduate Medical Education National Advisory Committee in September 1980, after four years of study, turned in to the United States Department of Health and Human Services a report announcing that there would soon be too many physicians. That report made "specific recommendations for federal control of a projected surplus of physicians."

"When has the modern U.S. federal bureaucracy neglected to issue regulations when an elite committee suggests such action? Seldom."

"The Image of the Health Insurance Industry." *Findings* (December 1990):

1–8.

The Health Insurance Association of America reported that less than 30% of Americans (27%) had a favorable view of the insurance industry (this is the insurance industry as a whole), whereas 64% of the same individuals had a favorable image of the computer industry, with only 36%ᵒ of Americans saying that they have a favorable impression of health insurers, 27% of liability insurers, 28% of auto insurers, and 43% of life insurers.

Indeed only 44% believed that the insurance industry meets its commitments, only 40% believe that it is responsible, only 43% believe it is helpful, only 37% believe that it solves problems, only 33% consider it trustworthy, 32% consider it truthful, 29% feel that the industry is fair, and only 27% feel that it is "caring."

Only 17% believe that medical insurance is affordable.

"Insurance Firms Get Jittery." *News-Leader* (21 July 1991): 1E.

The fourth major U.S. life insurance to fail this year, Mutual Benefit Life of New Jersey, was the subject of this article.

Of the top ten real estate lenders among U.S. insurers, number five was Principal Mutual Life with $11 billion in real estate holdings, or 46.3% of its assets.

Incidentally, Mutual Benefit was not a high flying junk bond excess investor.

"Insurer to Cover 12-Week Old's Heart Transplant." Springfield *News-Leader* (Friday, 22 June 1990).

Nationwide Insurance, the primary insurer, originally refused to pay the claim, but "negotiations" through an attorney and the Missouri Division of Insurance led them to pay the claim.

At the rate medical expenses are going, the total bill will change from $640 billion in 1990 to $1.5 trillion by 2000. Medical expenses represent up to 43% of corporate profits, and it is quite clear that the cost containment efforts of the past 21 years have not been significantly beneficial.

Probably a minimum of 80–85% of all medical expenses come from preventable lifestyle factors.

"IRS Employees Use Tax Money to Pump Iron." *News-Leader* (Sunday, 4 August 1991): 13A.

At the headquarters of the Internal Revenue Service in Washington, DC, bureaucrats use a health club at a cost to the American public of $525,000, and be aware that this is only for 125 employees! Typical government costs.

James, Frank E. "Study Lays Groundwork for Tying Health Costs to Workers' Behavior." *Wall Street Journal* (14 April 1987).

Prudential Insurance Company planned to market group insurance tied to health habits.

From 1980 to 1986, the percentage of employees who had to pay part of their medical insurance premiums increased from 25% to 41%.

Justice, Blair. *Who Gets Sick: Thinking and Health.* Houston: Peak Press, 1987.

Dr. Justice begins by documenting the remarkable ignorance of distinguished scientists about the effects of thoughts and motives upon the immune system. Perhaps a statement by Candice Pert, chair of the section on brain biochemistry of the National Institute of Mental Health, is worth repeating: "Scientific revolutions are very interesting. The way they happen is that most people may deny them and resist them. And then there's more and more of an explosion, and there's a paradigm shift" (p. 18).

Over and over again, Dr. Justice documents that stress "wrecks the immune system, gives people heart attacks, raises the risk of cancer," etc .

A very brief review of the 51-page bibliography of this more than 400-page book is worth giving because I know of no other work in which so much information about psychoneuroimmunology is summarized.

"Diet and nutrition appear to be related to the largest number of human cancers, tobacco smoking is related to about 30 to 40%" (p. 22).

"The more people perceive uncontrollable stress in their lives, the more they may turn to diets that place them at greater risk of cancer as well as heart disease" (p. 22). In other words, they eat more junk food.

"Disease is not so much the effect of noxious, external forces—the 'bugs,' both literal and figurative, in our lives—as it is the faulty efforts of our minds and bodies to deal with them" (p. 28).

"Illness or disease, then, occurs more from our vulnerability than from external agents that are the cause of our health problems. The more vulnerable we are, the more risk we run of getting sick" (p. 29).

"Our mind and behavior, our environment, and our genetic predispositions are the common contributors to disease" (p. 29).

"About one-fourth of the individuals experienced more than half of all the illnesses and over two-thirds of the total days of disability" (p. 34).

"Those who were more dissatisfied and discontented in general had more numerous illnesses" (p.34).

He emphasizes that those individuals who are most frequently ill have lower morale and much greater job dissatisfaction, as well as a greater perception of stress outside their lives. In other words, when we become ill, we have done something else which lowers our immunity.

There is considerable evidence that even such "simple" and relatively common childhood infections, streptococcal infections, and other respiratory illnesses, are approximately four times more frequent when families are in a situation which they consider stressful. Thus, emotional factors are critically important in "the activation of viruses as well as the body's ability to resist and contain such agents" (p. 38).

"There is always one system that, according to external influences or hereditary, is the weakest. It is the weak system that is first affected by stressors" (p. 40).

Even individuals who develop rheumatoid arthritis have the tendency towards this, measured by abnormal blood tests. They do not develop the rheumatoid arthritis as long as they are coping. When their coping skills fail, the rheumatoid arthritis manifests.

Actually it is not what most of us perceive as stress, but the way we react to stress, our perception of stress, our feeling of loss of control over the events of our lives, that seem to be the most significant factors. Even 2,400 years ago, Hippocrates felt that illness was the result of change. He included changes in seasons as well as other changes as major contributors to illness.

As early as 1910, "the famous British physician Sir William Osler devoted his Lumleian Lectures on angina pectoris to 'stress and strain'" (p. 48).

"Whether stress does us in depends largely on how we view our troubles and what chemical messages we trigger in our brains" (p.

52).

"A chronically hostile, cynical, or distrusting attitude can contribute to our risk of atherosclerosis and heart disease" (p. 53).

Selye talked about "choosing" the wrong reaction to an external event.

Suzanne Kobasa and associates of Chicago found that "the healthy managers considered change, good or bad, as an inevitable part of life and an opportunity for growth and new experience rather than as a threat to security" (p. 58).

"Those who stay healthy under stress, Kobasa found, have in addition to a sense of control and challenge, a commitment to life. They are deeply involved in their work and families, and this commitment gives them a sense of meaning, direction, and excitement" (p. 59).

Thus psychological "hardiness" is the result of a personal "belief in control, commitment, and challenge" (p. 60).

Interestingly, we can either adopt or reject that sense of belief on the sense of control. This is totally compatible with Viktor Frankl's concepts from *Man's Search for Meaning*, in which he stated that, although confined to a German concentration camp with remarkable abuse and indignity, the one thing that could not be taken from him was his "right to choose" his attitude.

"A study at Vanderbilt University showed that ego strength was the most powerful predictor of whether a person experienced acute illness and for how long" (p. 63).

In addition to actual illness itself, our abilities even to produce natural killer cells, the white blood cells that help destroy cancer and viruses, is strongly affected by our ability to cope. Those who cope better have higher levels of natural killer cell activity after immunization for swine flu. High anxiety and depression lower the activity of natural killer cells.

"It seems that the most hazardous health effects of anxiety, distress, anger, or depression may occur in people who already have lowered immune function" (p. 74).

Individuals who have a great need to control their environment give an artificially high impression of a higher incidence of upper respiratory illnesses and lower levels of certain types of immune antibodies.

"The more we perceive ourselves as being chronically hassled or experience negative moods, the more likely we will have lower levels of helper T-cells and greater susceptibility to some illnesses" (p. 76).

Norepinephrine, for instance, a primary stress chemical, blocks the ability of white blood cells to kill tumor cells.

"People who are cynical or have hostile attitudes or suppressed anger are found to have more atherosclerosis and blockage of coronary arteries" (p. 78).

This is totally compatible with Eysenck's work (see chapter 8).

Norepinephrine contributes to high blood pressure, hardening of the arteries, and even heart attacks; cortisone makes us more vulnerable to infections and cancer; low dopamine is associated with a lack of sense of pleasure and reward (p. 84).

On the other hand, an excess of dopamine is one of the findings in schizophrenia (p. 88).

I think probably one of the most interesting facts of all is that people with depression have excessive electrical activity in the right hemisphere. This has been published extensively and confirmed in our own clinic.

"When the neocortex of the right brain is removed, immune function is enhanced, apparently as a result of eliminating the source of depressive images. When the cortex of the left hemisphere is removed, T-cells are lost and immunity diminishes. Activation of the left brain is associated with optimism" (p. 104).

Thus, rational logical thinking does enhance both immune function and well-being.

There is an excellent chapter on "Mood, Food, and Pain" which is worth reading because Dr. Justice emphasizes the many interrelationships that occur between various amino acids and carbohydrates, as well as in how our bodies function both mentally and in the immune system.

" ... the quality of our relationships may have more to do with how often we get sick and how soon we get well than our genes, chemistry, diet, or environment" (p. 127).

Even tuberculosis is much more common in individuals who are both isolated and marginal "with little social support" (p. 128).

Those individuals who have less contact with family and friends and fewer social ties are much more prone to illness. Again, this is an excellent chapter emphasizing the tremendous importance of good interpersonal relationships.

Taking personal responsibility and having a positive outlook are two of the most critical factors in health. Even in a nursing home, those patients who are encouraged to take more self-responsibility have a death rate that is one-half that of individuals who are not pushed to take self-responsibility (within 18 months!) (p. 142).

Individuals who have more education, emotional support, and relaxation exercises have shorter hospital stays, faster recovery, and fewer complications (p. 145).

Relaxation skills enhance immunity (p. 158).

"Giving people something to care for can enhance their sense of control in life" (p. 258).

"Those who believed their health was excellent had one-third the risk of death than those who perceived their health was poor" (p. 265). This applies to individuals 65 years of age or older, and they were followed for six years.

"Work satisfaction and happiness were found to predict longevity better than any health or physical activity factor" (p. 266).

"The quality of a person's marriage, as he or she perceives it, has been found to be a more powerful predictor of happiness than even satisfaction with work or relationships with friends. Marital satisfaction is significantly associated with both level of immune function and psychological well-being" (p. 266).

"Some 30 double-blind studies have now concluded that Valium® (diazepam) is no more clinically effective than a placebo is for anxiety, which is the complaint the drug is most prescribed to relieve" (p. 289).

The pessimistic views of a doctor only exacerbate the helpless feelings of the patient" (p. 293).

"Greater intoxication from marijuana occurs when it is smoked among friends than strangers" (p. 297).

* When we receive a drug or a chemical, "the effects that we experience are the combined results of both the chemical contents of the substance and our beliefs" (p. 299).

"Halsted Holman, professor of medicine at Stanford University School of Medicine, argues that 'three of the four most commonly prescribed drugs treat no specific illness'" (p. 301).

"We have a choice, then, of teaching the brain to turn on healing systems or the opposite" (p. 326).

Keeler, Emmett, and John E. Rolph. "How Cost Sharing Reduced Med-

ical Spending of Participants in the Health Insurance Experiment."
JAMA 249:16 (22/29 April 1983): 2220–2.

"In a controlled trial of the effects of medical insurance on spending
and health status, much less was spent on medical care when patients
had to pay for it themselves. They economized by being less prone to
seek treatment or be hospitalized for their illnesses. The average cost
per hospitalization and per ambulatory episode was the same for all
insurance plans."

Keeler, Emmett B., et. al. *Effects of Cost Sharing on Physiological Health,
Health Practices, and Worry.* Santa Monica, CA: The Rand Corporation,
August 1987.

They mention the fact that they previously reported that patients
"with limited cost sharing had approximately one-third less use of
medical services, similar general self-assessed health, and worse
blood pressure, functional far vision, and dental health than those
with free care."

In the current study, using 20 additional measures of physiological
health with studies carried out on 3,565 adults, people who had cost
sharing scored better on 12 measures and worse only for functional
near vision. People with cost sharing had less worry and pain from
physiological conditions on 33 of 44 comparisons. Those with cost sharing fared worse on three types of cancer screening and better on weight,
exercise, and drinking. The bottom line ... "Except for patients with
hypertension or vision problems, the effects of cost sharing on health
were minor."

Kitagawa, Evelyn W., and Philip M. Hauser. *Differential Mortality in the
United States.* Cambridge: Harvard University Press, 1973.

The major areas of nonwhite mortality are New Jersey, Maryland,
Virginia, West Virginia, Kentucky, Tennessee, North Carolina, South
Carolina, Georgia, Alabama, and Mississippi. These are age-adjusted
death rates. Nevertheless, the highest white male mortality covered a
large portion of the south Atlantic seaboard and the Gulf Coast.
Regions of lowest white female mortality included the Southern
Piedmont, and the highest for white women included the Rocky
Mountain subregion and the southern New Mexico region, as well as
the southern Lake Michigan industrial area. Metropolitan areas, in
general, have much higher mortality rates than rural areas. For non-
whites in general, death rates were 48% higher for females and 25%
higher for males.

The other conclusions are that the greater amount of education individuals have, the longer they live. The higher median family income is, the longer people live. For instance, white females with one year or more of college live an average of 10 years longer than those with less than five years of school. Among white males, the increase is only 3.2 years for the college educated men vs. those with less than five years of school. From another point of view, among white females 25 and older, the mortality ratio was 78% higher with less than five years of school than for those who had completed four years of college.

Klarman, Herbert E. "Observations on Health Care Technology: Measurement, Analysis, and Policy." In Stuart H. Altman and Robert Blendon (eds.). *Medical Technology: The Culprit Behind Health Care Costs* (proceedings of the 1977 Sun Valley Forum on National Health). Washington: United States Department of Health, Education, and Welfare; U.S. Government Printing Office, 282, 287.

"More recently, in the Marshfield, Wisconsin, group practice clinic, as reported by Joel Broida, conversion of part of the clientele fee-for-service to a prepayment plan did not result in any saving in hospital use; a possible explanation is that the hospital beds were still there to be used."

The author concluded, "One-sixth of the increase in expenditures for short-term hospital care in the decade 1966–76 is due to a rise in utilization ... Five-sixths of the increase is due to the increasing costs per adjusted patient day."

Knowles, John H. Winter. "The Responsibility of the Individual." Cambridge, MA: *Daedalus, The Journal of the American Academy of Arts and Sciences,* 1977.

"More than half the reduction in mortality rates over the past three centuries occurred before 1900 and was due in nearly equal measure to improved nutrition and in reduced exposure to air- and water-borne infection" (p. 57).

" ... over 99% of us are born healthy and made sick as a result of personal misbehavior and environmental conditions. The solution to the problems of ill health in modern American society involves individual responsibility, in the first instance, and social responsibility through public legislative and private voluntary efforts, in the second instance. Alas, the medical profession isn't interested, because the intellectual, emotional, and financial rewards of the present system are too great and because there is no incentive and very little demand to change" (p.

58).

"Prevention of disease means foresaking the bad habits which many people enjoy—overeating, too much drinking, taking pills, staying up at night, engaging in promiscuous sex, driving too fast, and smoking cigarettes—or, put another way, it means doing things which require special effort—exercising regularly, going to the dentist, practicing contraception, insuring a harmonious family life, submitting to screening examinations" (p. 59).

" ... the next major advances in the health of the American people will come from the assumption of individual responsibility for one's own health and a necessary change in habits for the majority of Americans" (p. 60).

"A large percentage of deaths (estimates up to 80%) due to cardiovascular disease and cancer are 'premature' that is, occur in relatively young individuals and are related to the individual's bad habits" (p. 62).

"Studies indicate that up to 80% of serious physical illnesses seem to develop at a time when the individual feels helpless or hopeless" (p. 62).

Kramsch, Dieter, M., et. al. "Reduction of Coronary Atherosclerosis by Moderate Conditioning Exercise in Monkeys on an Atherogenic Diet." *New England Journal of Medicine* 305:25 (17 December 1981): 1483–9.

Overall, exercise was associated with substantially reduced overall atherosclerotic involvement. It also produced larger hearts and wider coronary arteries, which further reduced the degree of narrowing of the arteries.

"Our data suggests that moderate exercise may prevent or retard coronary heart disease in primates."

Lacombe, Michael A. "Social Darwinism." *JAMA* 260:19 (18 November 1988): 2907.

"The system cannot run on the present budget. Those are the cold facts."

"You pile on meetings and committees and politics and forms and the hassles with Medicare and Medicaid, and you just can't do a good job.

So I'm sorry. I'm going to try something else."

Lanning, Joyce A. "Are Medical Education Dollars Buying What They Should?" *JAMA* 238 (12 September 1977): 1153–7.

The article reports that Flexner in his famous report of medical education in 1910 did not look at the quality of care that the patient receives "but sought to improve it indirectly by emphasizing the quality of medical education ... Almost 70 years later, we are still grappling with ways of more directly measuring quality of care."

"This brings up the setting and focus of medical care, or the dilemma of sick cure vs. health care ... But in our enchantment with the sick-cure possibilities of modern medicine, and the technological imperative (if you know it can be done, do it), we have tended to overlook the other determinants of health."

"History shows the most dramatic improvements in the health of our people as a group have been from cleaning up the water supply: sanitation, not medical care. Next in importance has been food: improved nutrition. Immunization comes in third ... The American Association for Advancement of Science estimates that 80 to 90% of all cancer in the United States is environmentally induced."

They quote a study which states that 50% of all life lost prematurely in Canada was the result of just a few health habits.

The author states that more than 90% of every health dollar is spent on the sick person.

"There is concern that the public is attempting to lay all the ills of society at the feet of physicians ... Many citizens like their own physician, but distrust other physicians."

"The research medical model for medical schools set up by Flexner has been highly successful in increasing our knowledge and understanding of disease, and has developed some expensive technologies to implement that knowledge. But it has not paid much attention to preventing disease or positively promoting physical and moral well-being."

As early as 1970 the Carnegie Commission on Higher Education questioned continuing emphasis on medical science. The author, Joyce Lanning, suggests that if physicians "cannot be expected to directly solve the broader health problems of society, they can at least refrain from being obstructionist as others, including patients, work to alter an environment that puts people at risk and to activate each person in his own behalf."

Lasagna, Louis. "Rationing Human Life." (editorial) *JAMA* 249:16 (22/29 April 22/29): 2223–5.

"In 1929, the United States spent 3.5% of its gross national product on health care. This had increased to 5.3% by 1960 and was an astonishing 10.3% by 1982."

"Or is it fair for one healthy person to require virtually no cost for health through a full life while another may assume a quarter of a million, a million, 5 million dollars of funds derived in some way from the public wealth to maintain one life?"

Dr. Lundberg, the editor of the journal, stated, "One thing is certain. Reality cannot be delayed. Not to decide is to decide."

It is now 20 years later and we have not decided.

Layle, John. "Why Health Costs Aren't Really Rising." *Missouri Internist* (May/June through November/December 1989).

Dr. Layle argues that the major "illusions" of medical costs have been created by inflation and that inflation was created not by doctors or hospitals, but in Washington by politicians and economists. He argued it cannot be cured "by peer review, pre-certification, second opinions, fee freezes, rationing, prospective payment, capitation, certification-of-need laws, or any other provider-targeted program."

Inflation results from over-production of money and/or the under-production of valuable goods and services. He argues that the American public is regularly misinformed or disinformed "by those persons and institutions usually held responsible for social enlightenment."

Dr. Layle uses a bar graph which shows the following changes between 1967 and 1978. Increased costs ... gold wedding ring, 400%; Levi jeans, 240%; one pound of hamburger, 150%; an appendectomy, 125%; a week in a semi-private hospital room, 150%.

Dr. Layle goes on to state, *"After correction for inflation,* health expenditures for 1981 through 1983 increased 4.6%, which was exactly the average annual rate of real growth for the preceding decade."

He emphasizes that most of the time graphs and charts show "unreal health expenditures distored by" inflation. He emphasized that both *Time* and *Newsweek* "selectively reported only the inflation-distorted change in prices of specific health services, thereby encouraging the illusion of 'skyrocketing' health costs."

Virtually invariably, the government, *Time*, *Newsweek*, and other media moguls have demonstrated increased medical or disease costs without correcting both for inflation and population growth. For instance, in the 20-year period between 1967 and 1987, the population of the country increased approximately 25%; that is, from 200 million to almost 250 million.

In a brilliant chart, the authors show that when we measure the United States health cost in constant dollars and corrected for population growth and then compare that with the subpopulations of high health care consumers who "have increased much more rapidly than subpopulations of low consumers," we see that the real increase in cost is not in excesses of the medical profession, but in the increased use of medical facilities. For instance, "Since the inception of Medicare (July 1, 1966), it's rolls have increased by 72%—from 18.8 million to 32.4 million, while the total population increased only 24%." It is well known that "health care requirements of older people up to age 85 is progressively higher than it is for younger people."

The authors go on to explain that "the illusion of 'skyrocketing health costs' has occurred largely because 'health care' has come to mean much more than health care. 'Health care' nowadays has two components: health producing costs such as bedside care; and non-health producing costs such as the cost of insurance, financing, borrowing, marketing, monitoring, planning, accounting, competing, electing, politicizing, compensating, and so forth." He estimates that at least 22% of the personal disease expenditures goes just to pay for the paper shuffling of the health bureaucracy. We now spend more than three times as much on bureaucracy as we did on all health care for every man, woman, and child in the United States in 1961! Indeed, Dr. Layle even goes on to explain that such costs as "television rental, educational programs, or sales through a gift shop or cafeteria" are exaggerated into disease costs today. It also includes such things as treatment of "ugliness," that is, such things as toupees, Rogaine® for hair growth, and plastic surgery for breast implants and other such things.

Lewis, Marlo, and Thomas Schatz. "Critical Government Waste Issues for the 102nd Congress." *Government Waste Watch* (Summer 1991): 14.

"During the past two years, federal domestic spending has increased more than twice as fast as the rate of inflation."

"Federal domestic spending has grown by 10% per year since 1989."

"Total federal spending now consumes more than 25% of the gross national product (GNP)—the highest level since 1946 and up from 22.3% in 1989."

Lewis, Richard. "California May Deregulate Physicians." *American Medical News* (18 July 1981): 1, 17.

Reports state that the California Board of Medical Quality Assurance was considering a radical proposal to deregulate the medical profession. The only exceptions would be that surgery and prescriptions for dangerous drugs would be restricted to physicians. Supposedly this would lead to less government intervention and fewer restrictions on individual freedoms, but of course it didn't happen and things probably have gotten more bureaucratic rather than less.

The State Medical Society of Wisconsin in its Medical Green Sheet, January 1978, stated, "A recent study by the University of Chicago shows that 61% of Americans think there is a crisis in health care—at least for other people. However, only 12% say they are generally dissatisfied with the health care they themselves receive. The causes of dissatisfaction most frequently cited were high costs and long amounts of time spent in waiting rooms."

Lillard, Lee A., et. al. *Preventive Medical Care: Standards, Usage, and Efficacy.* Santa Monica, CA: The Rand Corporation, August 1986.

They found no statistically significant effect on a randomly assigned physical examination upon either the use of health services or health status three years later.

Their data show "that preventive care does not respond significantly to out-of-pocket costs, but is less responsive to cost sharing than is nonpreventive care."

In their study only one-fourth of men had any use of "preventive services." Two-thirds of women received recommended Pap smears, but very few received mammograms. Less than half of children 18 months and younger received recommended polio and DPT.

Madigan, Francis C. "Role Satisfaction and Length of Life in a Closed Population." American Journal of Sociology 67 (May 1962): 640–9.

This paper reported on a large American subdivision of an order of Roman Catholic priests. It reports that they enjoyed a more favorable mortality experience than white males of the general population for comfortable years, which suggests that high role satisfaction is related to favorable mortality experience. These individuals smoked an average amount, had a high cholesterol diet, less exercise than the general population, and more prevalent obesity, and yet from 45–74 years of age their mortality rate was only 86% that of the general population. They attribute this to the degree of satisfaction, but didn't mention the three hours a day of meditation. They do mention regularity of life and that they are more intelligent.

Manson, JoAnn, et. al. "Body Weight and Longevity: A Reassessment." *JAMA* 257:3 (16 January 1987): 353–8.

The major conclusion is that the minimum mortality occurs at relative weights at least 10% below the United States average, and of course the most striking change being that the mortality ratio for smokers, both in men and women, is approximately twice that of nonsmokers.

Mark, Vernon. "A Prescription for the Rising Cost of Medical Care." *JAMA* 237:22 (30 May 1977): 2383–4.

Dr. Vernon Mark suggested that solutions include, among other things, an increase in specialty training; consolidation of sophisticated centers for elective surgery and deep X-ray therapy; and a greater emphasis of specialists as consultants and less participation in primary management.

Markle, George B. "We Physicians are Fiduciary Failures." *JAMA* 239 (21 April 1978): 1629–30.

The author stated that physicians "are in a position to bankrupt him (the patient) or the society that pays for his care."

McNerney, Walter J. "Control of Health-Care Costs in the 1980's." *New England Journal of Medicine* 303:19 (6 November 1980): 1088–95.

The author indicates that "for approximately 20 years there has been growing public concern over the cost and accessibility of health services."

He mentions "10,000 pages of Medicare pronouncements."

"Clearly government programs have not worked well."

He doesn't mention that he is part of the cause—an officer at Blue Cross Blue Shield.

"Medicine: Transplant or Tuneup." *New Sense Bulletin* 16:10 (July 1991): 1, 7.

"Has the point of no return been reached for the collapsing health care system in the United States?"

"Editor-in-Chief George Lundberg of the *Journal of the American Medical Association* is sure that it has. In the midst of what he termed an 'aura of inevitability,' Lundberg decided well over a year ago that the entire May 15, 1991, issue of the Journal would be devoted to the crisis."

"Most of the *JAMA* proposals entail keeping and improving upon certain aspects of the American system as opposed to scrapping it in favor of the Canadian model—simple surgery, not a transplant. But it is easy to doubt that mere tinkering with such an anarchic system can settle the crisis."

"Men: Exercise, Save Your Life." *USA Today* (20 November 1986): 1D.

Men can lower their risks of dying from a heart attack more than fourfold by getting more physical exercise.

Mills, Jeffrey. "AMA Practices Restraint, Competition, Judge Rules." *LaCrosse Tribune* (Wednesday, 29 November 1978).

This article was on the Federal Trade Commission's injunction against the AMA for enforcing a "code of ethics" that "banned physician solicitation of business, severely restricted physician advertising, and took other steps that constituted unfair methods of competition."

Missouri Drug Utilization Review Report 3:1 (August 1991).

"A significant number of drugs in common daily use can actually cause depression?"

They state that depressive symptoms may occur in 13–20% of the population, as many as 20–35% of elderly patients are depressed, and the lifetime prevalence of depression is about 15%.

The following drugs are listed as being associated with depression:

Antihypertensives
 clonidine/methylodopa
 Guanethidine
 Hydralazine
 indapamide
 reserpine
 prazosin
Appetite Suppressants
 amphetamines

fenfluramine
phenmetrazine

Antiarthritics
phenylbutazone
idomethacin

Antianxiety
benzodiazepines
meprobamate
chloral hydrate
barbiturates
sedative hypnotics

Antipsychotics
phenothiazines
fluphenazine
haloperidol
thioxanthenes

Analgesics
opiates
pentazocine

Anticonvulsants
succinate derivatives
barbiturates
carbamazepine

Antiparkinsonians
amantadine
L-dopa
bromocriptine

Cardiovascular
digitalis
procainamide

Antimicrobials
cycloserine
ethambutol
metronidazole

Miscellaneous
alcohol
choline
disulfiram
physostigmine

lecithin
antineoplastic agents
cimetidine/ranitidine

Organic Pesticides

Mitka, Mike. "Cost Frequency of St. Paul Claims Up in '90." *American Medical News* (5 August 1991): 11.

The frequency of claims per 100 physicians in 1984 was 16.4, in 1985 it was 17.9. It dipped to 12.4 per 100 physicians in 1989, and climbed to 13.6 in 1990.

St. Paul Fire and Marine Insurance is the largest medical liability insurance, with 30,000 physicians in 42 states.

The average cost of reported claims rose to $36,400 in 1990 from $32,700 in 1989.

Mitka, Mike. "Cost of Physician Services Up Only Slightly So Far in '91." *American Medical News* (12 August 1991): 13–4.

"For the 12 months ended in June, hospital room prices increased 10.1% and prescription drugs rose 8%."

The annualized inflation rate for June was 2.7%; physician services, 2.9%; overall medical care, 7.8%; hospital room prices, 8.5%; and prescription drug prices, 11.5%.

"More U.S. Adults are Getting Less Sleep, Study Says." *American Medical News* (1 August 1, 1986): 22.

Apparently only approximately 12% of individuals were getting a regular amount of sleep in 1983. He reported that between 1977 and 1983 unfavorable health practices increased in lack of sleep, lack of eating breakfast, snacking, decreased physical activity, alcohol consumption, and body weight.

Mullen, Patrick. "Blues PPO in Mo. Asks Hospitals for a Cash Donation." *Health Week* (12 June 1989): 14, 33.

Blue Cross Blue Shield of Kansas City was asking local hospitals to help them make up for their $28.3 million loss in the previous year.

Newhouse, Joseph P., et. al. "Some Interim Results From a Controlled Trial of Cost Sharing in Health Insurance." New England Journal of

Medicine 305:25 (17 December 1981): 1501–7.

In a study of 7,706 persons participating in a controlled trial of alternative health-insurance policy, "interim results indicate that persons fully covered for medical services spend about 50% more than do similar persons with income-related catastrophy insurance. Full coverage leads to more people using services and to more services per user."

Ng, Lorenz, et. al. "The Health Promotion Organization: A Practical Intervention Designed to Promote Healthy Living." *Public Health Reports* 93:5 (September-October 1978): 446–55.

The authors state that the leading causes of morbidity and premature death are associated with living patterns. For example, heart attack, cancer, accidents, and strokes are associated with living patterns.

The authors propose the development of a Health Promotion Organization to reward healthy lifestyles, teach techniques that promote health, and stimulate more effective linkages between private sector and government.

"Private insurance companies presently reward sickness, while the proposed HPO will encourage the private sectors to shift its incentives from illness to health."

They recommend that "the well, the worried well, and the asymptomatic sick would be offered education and skill training in self-care and self-help."

Nuprin Pain Report. Washington: National Academic Press, 1985.

The *Nuprin Pain Report* was the first broadly based systematic study of frequency, severity, and costs associated with pain in adults 18 years of age or older. The most common pain problem was headache. Seventy-three per cent of Americans have one or more a year; 56% have backache one or more days per year; 51% have joint pain one or more days per year; 46% have stomach pain one or more days per year; premenstrual syndrome occurs in 40% of all women and dental pain in 27% of all Americans.

Four billion work days are lost per year because of pain with an average of 23 work days for every person in the United States.

Only 16% of Americans say that they never feel stressed; 46% say that they feel stressed one or more days per week.

Persons with headache, premenstrual pain, and stomach pain all believe the single most important cause is stress.

Those individuals who exercise three or more days per week, who do not smoke, drink little alcohol, and do not watch television have significantly less pain.

Smokers have much more stomach pain. Drinkers have more headache and stomach pain. Heavy TV watchers have more headache, back ache, and joint pain.

Of those with more than just occasional pain, 50% see a physician, 18% see a chiropractor, 12% see a pharmacist, 3% see a pain specialist or nutritionist, and 2% see an acupuncturist or spiritual faith healer.

Of those who saw an M.D., the M.D. prescribed a prescription drug 42% of the time, a non-prescription drug 17% of the time, exercise 18% of the time, diet 10% of the time, heat and cold therapy 9% of the time, meditation and relaxation 7% of the time, hypnosis none of the time, TENS only 2% of the time, and biofeedback only 1% of the time.

Individuals who saw physicians perceived that they achieved relief 70% of the time; with a chiropractor they achieved relief 90% of the time; when they saw a nutritionist they received relief 69% of the time; they received relief from a dentist 67% of the time; and they received relief from a specialist 65% of the time.

Thirty-eight per cent of individuals with headache had it between 6 and 100 days per year; 27% had back pain 6 to 100 days per year; 27% had muscle pain 6 to 100 days per year; 24% had joint pain the same length of time; 18% had stomach pain; 28% of women had premenstrual problems 6–100 days per year; and 8% had dental pain.

Forty-six per cent of all women had premenstrual pain an average of 11 days per year.

Forty-nine per cent of individuals had medium to high stress. High stress increases the incidence of pain by approximately 50%.

Of those who had pain six or more days per year, 30–50% lost sleep because of it. Of those who had pain six or more days per year, 23–59% found that the pain was severe to unbearable (7–10 on a scale of 0–10).

Twenty-five per cent of the people surveyed did no significant physical exercise at all; 70% of smokers do no significant physical exercise.

Of the pain sufferers, 43% saw a physician once or not at all in the last year; 19%, twice; 10%, three times; 28%, four or more times.

O'Dell, Kathleen. "Health Care Costs Going Up, Up, UP." Springfield *News-Leader* (Friday, 3 November 1989): sec. D.

"Sixty percent of the respondents (? Missouri) increasingly feel employee contributions are not keeping pace with medical care costs."

"The requirement to receive a second surgical opinion has not been proven to be cost effective, and most of the surgeries are done any-way."

"Employers have seen an explosion in the demand for psychiatric/substance abuse benefits, but 56% aren't sure if the programs are actually saving any money in production time or absenteeism."

"Employers increased the benefits for outpatient surgeries, and now those benefits are costing 10% more than inpatient procedures."

Ornish, Dean, et. al. "Effects of Stress Management Training and Dietary Changes in Treating Ischemic Heart Disease." JAMA 249:1 (7 January 1983,): 54–9.

Patients who were given stress management instruction and relaxation exercises, meditation, and a vegan diet with minimal amounts of non-fat yogurt in the diet, also excluding salt, sugar, alcohol, and caffeine, showed a 44% mean increase in duration of exercise, a 55% mean increase in total work performed, a 25% mean decrease in plasma cholesterol, and a 91.0% decrease in frequency of anginal episodes.

Paffenbarger, Ralph S., et. al. "A Natural History of Athleticism and Cardiovascular Health." *JAMA* 252:4 (27 July 1984): 491–5.

Habitual post-college exercise, not student sports play, predicts low coronary heart disease risk. Exercise benefit is independent of smoking, obesity, weight gain, hypertension, and adverse parental disease history.

Page, Irvine H. "Science, Intuition, and Medical Practice." *Post-Graduate Medicine* 64 (November 1978): 217–21.

"Much of the medical practice should be based on the application of intuition rather than of science."

"No society has ever thrived for centuries without a transcendent belief in something greater than itself."

Palmer, Barbara. "Firms Try to Crack Back Problems." *USA Today* (Monday, 22 July 1985): 1B–2B.

> Back problems affect approximately 75 million Americans, with 2.5 million adults totally disabled. There are approximately 200,000 surgical procedures per year (some statistics say up to 450,000!). The cost to industry from absenteeism and disability is $14 billion a year. It is the second leading cause of hospitalization after pregnancy. It is responsible for 18 million doctor visits a year and costs about 93 million workdays annually (among those still working).

Pelletier, Kenneth. "A Review and Analysis of the Health and Cost-Effective Outcome Studies of Comprehensive Health Promotion and Disease Prevention Programs." *American Journal of Health Promotion* 5:4 (March/April 1991): 311–3.

> "Given the limitations and caveats cited above, there is a clear and growing body of evidence indicating that comprehensive health promotion programs are both health and cost-effective."

Perrone, Janice. "Blues Plan Failure Staggers West Virginia: Doctors Wonder About Future of State's Care." *American Medical News* (2 November 1990): 1, 27.

> Only 27% of the physicians in that state were committed to staying in the state when a survey was done following this problem.

Peters, Tom. "Save Time, Money by Loving Your Customers." *News-Leader* (Monday, 22 July 1991): 3D.

> He quotes Dr. Kerr White, retired Deputy Director for Health Sciences at the Rockefeller Foundation, stating, "Between 40 and 60% of all therapeutic benefits (from contemporary clinical interventions) can be attributed to a combination of the placebo and Hawthorne effects, two code words for caring and concern, or what most people call 'love.'"

Petersdorf, Robert G. "Sounding Board—Academic Medicine: No Longer Threadbare or Genteel." *New England Journal of Medicine* 304:14 (2 April 1981): 841–3.

> As early as 1981 Robert G. Petersdorf, M.D., stated in "Sounding Board" in *JAMA*, "Patient care is also less satisfying than it used to be. In the first place, there is more of it, and secondly, it has become

more bureaucratized. We stamp, initial, and sign notes for the sake of complying with regulations."

Petersdorf, Robert G. "In Defense of Medicine." *Pharos* (Summer 1991): 2–7.

The author believes that "things are not as grim as they have been depicted."

The "crest" of the percentage of applicants for medical school was 1974. By 1988 the applicant pool had declined by more than one-third. He quotes some interesting things to account for that. Twenty-five new medical schools opened in the 70s, while the size of the entering class increased from 11,500 to more than 17,000.

He mentions more than 6,000 heart transplants in the United States "because the public wants them."

"Physician's Opinion Survey Report: Part One." *Leaders' Letter* (a newsletter of the State Medical Society of Wisconsin) 1:41 (12 November 1976).

This report states, "In Wisconsin, 85% of the physicians feel they have little clout with the politicians. Eighty-four percent cite high concerns over the cost of professional liability insurance. Eighty percent are concerned about third party intrusion into a physician's professional judgment."

Fifty-one per cent of the physicians either did not like or strongly did not like the value they received from the AMA.

Twenty per cent of the physicians stated that they worked 40–50 hours per week; 36%, 50–60 hours; 25%, 60–70 hours; 8%, 70–80 hours; and 5% indicated they worked more than 80 hours per week.

Praiss, Israel, and Craig Gjerde. "Cost Containment Through Medical Education." *JAMA* 244:1 (4 July 1980): 53–5.

In 1971 the authors report that data from the Social Security bulletins indicated that in 1971 hospital care took up 35.8% of all medical expenses; in 1973, 38.8%; and in 1978, 40.4%. Physicians received in 1971, 20% ; 1973, 18.4%; and in 1978, 19.8%. Nursing home care in the same years took up 3.8% in 1971, 4.2% in 1973, and 7.8% in 1978. Interestingly, drugs and drug sundries took up 10.9% in 1971, 9.5% in 1973, and only 7.7% in 1978.

Private Practice 29 (May 1988): 1.

An average of 65,793 people see the Bears play every Sunday, but doctors see 45 times that many patients every day, namely 3 million patients per day.

Promoting Health in America: Breakthroughs and Harbingers. Battlecreek, MI: W. K. Kellogg Foundation, 1989.

"By the mid-1970's the time was right to begin widespread efforts to stimulate changes in personal lifestyle that promised an improved state of health" (p. 11).

Several large-scale studies, stretching back 20 years prior to that "had shown an association between the major causes of death and disability, on the one hand, and selected patterns of addictive behaviors (e.g., use of alcohol, tobacco, and drugs), poor diet, and lack of exercise, on the other" (p. 11).

They go on to discuss techniques for analyzing the results of poor habits leading to "premature" disease or death.

They cite such statistics as tobacco use being the major cause of premature death, "accounting for some 338,022 deaths in 1980 alone," but they talk about high blood pressure causing 297,162 "needless deaths," and *overnutrition* causing 289,502 deaths. "These three risk factors together accounted for 73.5% of the preventable causes of death." Overnutrition is defined as "excess ingestion of salt, cholesterol, and fatty foods, obesity, and the like" (p. 16).

Interestingly, the leading risk factor in the United States, as determined by the potential years of life lost before age 65, is injury not due to alcohol, which is 1.8 million cumulative years; alcohol and tobacco use each account for 1.5 million years of potential years of life lost before age 65; unintended pregnancy leads to 520,000 potential years lost before age 65; handguns to 350,683 years; inadequate access to health and medical care to 324,709 years; and gaps in health screening to 172,793 years (p. 16).

As a result of these kinds of factors, the Kellogg Foundation sponsored some pilot projects to help educate individuals to the benefits of adopting healthy habits and behavioral changes. Out of some worksite programs came some interesting findings. For instance, just getting this information into any company requires "a high level of commitment from management and the workers who will be the foci of the program" (p. 29). It takes a fair amount of time to "recruit" employees to participate.

Interestingly, they demonstrated that "blue collar workers are as interested in health promotion programs as white collar workers, if the programs are developed to allow participation during or aligned with the workday" (p. 29).

They also showed that health promotion could be as effective in small companies as in large ones (p. 29).

In one study they report that for 4.75 years after an educational behavioral program was introduced, "participants averaged 24% lower health costs than nonparticipants. The imputed savings in health care costs exceeded program costs for this cohort by a factor of 1.45" (p. 32).

They talk about the fact that fewer than 1,000 of the 16,000 school districts in the United States have introduced a comprehensive approach to school health education (p. 33),

In another program for low-income individuals in Texas, they found among program participants that there was a 3% weight reduction, 8% less smoking; 9% less alcohol consumption among the men, but not among the women; 18% increase in daily exercise among men, and 20% among women; a 13% reduction in the indices of stress among men, and 19% among women (p. 45).

They emphasize the serious lack of adequate training among health professionals. They mention the fact that very little multidisciplinary continuing professional education is available, that nationally only 70 physicians are pursuing post-graduate training in occupational medicine, despite the fact that 100,000 workers die each year from job-related diseases and there are 400,000 new cases of occupational disease each year as of 1982. Furthermore, one out of every eight industrial workers is injured on the job. Overall, occupational disease is the fourth most frequent cause of death, exceeded only by heart disease, cancer, and stroke. They emphasize the need for comprehensive interdisciplinary models of training among health professionals, including generalists and specialists in medicine, nursing, industrial hygiene, and all allied health professionals (pp. 73–4).

"Psychiatric Disorders Affect 20%." *The Daily News* (3 October 1984) 3A.

Twenty-nine million Americans at that time had "mental illness."

"Reagan OK's Health Plan." *The Daily News* (Friday, 13 February 1987): 1A-2A.

"According to a Gallup poll, three out of four Americans misunderstood how far the Medicare program and retirement health care insurance will carry them."

"Medicare covers only 30–40% of expenses." That's the bottom line, folks.

Reed, Ralph R., and Daryl Evans. "A Deprofessionalism of Medicine: Causes, Effects, and Responses." *JAMA* 258:22 (11 December 1987): 3279, 3282.

The authors state that there is great anxiety among physicians because of "the reduction of physician prerogatives in the delivery of health care. The precipitous drop in the professional autonomy of physicians is alarming if one believes that professionalism still provides the best model of health care delivery in terms of benefits to patients and society."

Rennie, Drummond. "Home Dialysis and the Costs of Uremia." *New England Journal of Medicine* 298 (16 February 1978): 399–400.

Just prior to 1972 the Social Security benefits were increased to extend Medicare coverage for chronic renal failure to almost the entire population of the United States. Within six years there were 37,000 patients having dialysis, with projections that this number would increase by about 50% within six to seven years.

Robin, Eugene D. *Matters of Life and Death: Risks vs. Benefits of Medical Care.* New York: W.H. Freeman & Company, 1984.

Dr. Robin, professor of medicine and physiology at Stanford University School of Medicine since 1970, a past president of the American Thoracic Society, a visiting professor of many medical schools, has been on the faculty at Harvard Medical School and the University of Pittsburgh and is a consultant to the National Institutes of Health and the VA.

Dr. Robin's book begins by stating that the remarkable accumulation of medical knowledge of the past 20 years "has been accompanied by a growing and unprecedented disillusionment with the application of this knowledge to patient care."

He states that he has certain assumptions:

- "The goal of doctors should be to help patients as much as possible (hardly a revolutionary or world-shattering assumption).
- Much of what we doctors do is tangential to that purpose.
- Much of what we do is harmful.

- Many of the tangential and harmful aspects of medical care could be changed.

- We doctors should take the major responsibility."

"Malpractice consists of a breech of the community's standards of medical practice. It occurs when a physician's activities do not conform to those practiced in the community. But suppose that most of the physicians in the community are wrong about some aspect of medical care. Then this systematic error represents the standard of medical care, and to conform to it is not malpractice."

He states, "You will be advised to consult doctors only when you believe that you are truly ill."

"This advice tends to slight an important function that doctors have assumed in our society: Dealing with patients whose main problem is an unhappy life. It is your privilege to consult a doctor for that purpose, but you should know that few doctors have high cure rates for unhappy lives, so that the chances of getting real help are small. Moreover, your visit may start a series of potentially dangerous medical tests and treatments."

He goes on to state that he believes it is "the system rather than individual doctors" who are "primarily responsible for the harm that patients may suffer."

He emphasizes that "the basic processes for introducing and using diagnostic and therapeutic measures in medicine contain serious flaws."

He states, "You will also learn that harmful practices introduced into medicine tend to proliferate and become epidemic."

He states that "retrospective clinical trials are notoriously unreliable."

He says, "Is it common practice in medicine to perform careful clinical trials before introducing tests that can affect the welfare of masses of patients? Sadly, the answer is No. This omission is one of the major systematic flaws in medicine. Incorrect medical practices do affect masses of patients."

"Chemotherapy with anti-cancer drugs prolongs the average total life span by perhaps 14 months. The treatment itself is associated with recurrent infections, fever, loss of appetite, and a series of other complications that make life miserable. During and after treatment, these patients require frequent rehospitalization. As a result, the actual prolongation of happy and productive life is considerably less than 14 months."

He goes on to describe the problems with human heart-lung transplantation. "This largely experimental procedure is being used for patients who are terminally ill with far-advanced disease of the blood vessels of the lung. To be successful, it requires the long-term use of a drug, cyclosporin-A, which has adverse effects on the kidneys and liver." He mentions that it also causes lymphoma in a higher percentage of patients.

"The high death rates for heart surgery in some medical centers are scandalous ... Little has been done to resolve this problem."

"Physicians frequently do not recognize that their inaccuracies may lead to management decisions that can harm their patients."

He believes that "physical examination is subject to greater observer error, leading to higher rates of false positives and false negatives."

He discusses such ridiculous diagnostic tests as brain biopsies to diagnose Alzheimer's disease, for which there is no satisfactory treatment. How can the "relatives or the patient benefit?"

He goes on to discuss other misuses of brain biopsies and concludes, "We may conclude that with rare exception the performance of brain biopsies stems from diagnostic zeal and makes little or no contribution to patient welfare. Brain biopsy in most circumstances is therefore an example of a systematic error in medical management."

"In spite of its inaccuracies, the routine use of ultrasound tests on all or most pregnant women has been advocated by some specialists."

He summarizes:

- "Many doctors have unrealistic estimates of how diagnostic methods of treatment may affect their patients.

- Diagnosis and treatment are often uncoupled and treatment and a happy outcome are often uncoupled.

- Much of medical testing is predictably tangential to the welfare of the patient and some results in harm. In some circumstances, this is unavoidable; in others, it is avoidable."

"The alarming factor is that, for most tests in medicine, we have no acceptable information on either diagnostic efficiency or therapeutic efficiency."

Dr. Robin believes that if you are truly sick, you'd better go to a medical doctor. He also states, "If you are not very sick, but need emotional support, you will surely find among doctors at least as many compassionate, sensitive, helpful humans as you will find in the alternative forms of health care."

Dr. Robin quotes one very large-scale study of 808 consecutive admissions to a university hospital medical ward. Roughly one-third of the patients admitted had developed either a major or minor complication associated with treatment. In 8% of the patients these were major complications, defined as mishaps that were potentially life threatening. In 2% of the patients, the iatrogenic episode contributed directly to the patient's death.

He mentioned that in several health care systems outside the United States the rate of hospitalization per unit of population is approximately one-half that of the United States.

He concludes that "you should agree to hospitalization only when you are seriously ill, or when you require the facilities of a hospital for treatment." In other words, you don't need to be in the hospital for diagnostic testing unless you are extremely ill.

Dr. Robin emphasizes some iatroepidemics; that is, epidemics induced by physicians. These include the use of Diethylstilbestrol to prevent spontaneous abortion and of course it led to a severe problem of early genital cancer and perhaps decreased fertility in those offspring; high oxygen exposure in premature infants leading to blindness; the use of Biguanidines, an oral drug for diabetes which causes sometimes fatal lactic acidosis; internal mammary artery ligation for coronary artery disease, which was used extensively with some deaths and considerable pain disability, and no value in improving or prolonging life; exercise radionuclide studies, with the result of "masses of patients undergoing an invasive procedure—coronary angiography—and, occasionally, bypass surgery"; ileal bypass in obesity, which results in liver disease, arthritis, and even death; Chloramphenicol in bone marrow depression, an antibiotic agent which can be very useful in extremely life threatening illnesses, but can also cause death; tonsilectomy in children, which is the most common procedure in children, but has been demonstrated to be of no general benefit in preventing chronic ear infections or recurrent throat infections; psychosurgery for schizophrenia, after which thousands of patients are made more disabled than ever; pneumothorax for tuberculosis in which the lung was collapsed and not only didn't help the tuberculosis, but greatly aggravated disability; adrenalectomy and sympathectomy for high blood pressure, in neither case did patients benefit from these procedures and some died; thyroid removal or suppression for coronary disease or chronic lung disease;

superficial femoral vein ligation for pulmonary embolism; immuno-suppressive leukemia agents being used for bronchial asthma and certain skin diseases; flow-directed catheters in blood vessels of the lung, "despite the fact that the measurements are of no real value in improving the treatment for most of these patients"; gastrojejunos-tomy for peptic ulcer; subtotal gastrectomy for peptic ulcers; Thalido-mide; radiation for acne, leading to a high incidence of skin cancer; radiation for status thymaticus, with a disease which never really existed and which led to cancer of the thyroid gland; radiation for ankylosing spondylitis, which led to a tenfold increase in leukemia, as well as local cancer, and was of no value; brain damage in new-borns from the use of Hexachlorophene antiseptic soap; a severe visual impairment and degeneration of the spinal cord with more than 10,000 cases of death from the use of Entero-Vioform, used to treat amoebic dysentery; excess deaths in asthmatic children from drugs.

Dr. Robin goes on to state the leading gynecological journal in this country in 1969 recommended the uterus should be removed elec-tively in every woman past age 35 and that both ovaries should be removed because this would get rid of premenstrual tension and avoid the rare possibility of ovarian cancer. In 1976 it was still being debated and "data indicated that about 2 women per 1,000 hysterec-tomies died and about 350 per 1,000 suffered complications."

"Assuming that 75 million women are in those age groups, most of American life would rotate around the performance of hysterec-tomies. This would cause a minimum of 150,000 deaths in normal(?) women, and 25 million normal(?) women, or one-third the total, would have iatrogenic complications."

Interestingly, he quotes an article which emphasized that this would improve life expectancy by 73 days!

"In 1970, there were twice as many surgeons per capita in the United States and twice as much surgery ... On the contrary, almost every careful survey indicates that the United States has an excessive sup-ply of surgeons; furthermore, the surplus is increasing."

"Evidence shows that the amount of surgery increases as the number of surgeons increases."

Except for premature birth, and in patients who have had an over-dose of drugs that impair breathing, "there is no acceptable evidence that care in the ICU improves more lives than it harms."

He emphasizes that many patients are admitted to the ICU "for the purpose of prolonging the process of their dying, rather than for the purpose of prolonging their lives."

"It can be concluded that the ICU is not a good place to die gracefully."

"One study indicates that, in the critically ill, major complications of treatment—life threatening complications—develop in one-fifth to one-third of all patients."

"Of the numerous forms of treatment used in patients in the ICU, very few can be scientifically justified and almost none have been shown to improve patient outcome."

He quotes the study in England in which "the death rate was lowest among those treated at home!"

"If you are suspected of having a heart attack, try to spend as little time as possible in the CCU (cardiac care unit)." This is probably good advice even if you are a definite heart attack victim.

It seems that the most important point is to be sure that you get some intravenous magnesium in the occurrence of a heart attack, and this almost is never done.

"The World Health Organization concluded that none of the screening tests in common use during the 1960's met all of these requirements." These requirements were essentially that the screening tests might do something useful for patients to prevent illness or death and not cause harm.

"Available evidence suggests that general health examinations are not useful."

Actually only a few tests are really useful: periodic examinations of healthy children, periodic prenatal examinations, tests for congenital hypothyroidism, and phenylketonuria and galactosemia in newborns.

He goes on to talk about the problems of a false positive as well as a false negative in the most commonly prescribed "preventive" screening test, the Pap smear. "The evidence indicating the benefit of Pap smears is derived from studies that were not controlled and is without supporting data on the number and the fate of the false positives."

He does think that the Pap smear may be useful if one has symptoms suggesting cancer such as vaginal bleeding at any abnormal time.

He quotes one study in which "there was disagreement among ten experts as to the presence or absence of cancer cells in about 40% of the specimens. In another study, in about two-thirds of the subjects, two Pap smears taken simultaneously from the same woman showed different results—no cancer in one sample and cancer in the other."

"Even without precise statistics, we can be certain that large numbers of normal subjects have been harmed by Pap testing."

He states you don't have to feel guilty if you decide not to have a Pap smear annually or on any kind of regular basis. Basically he thinks you should have the test only when you have abnormal symptoms.

Dr. Robin goes on to discuss the problems of mass screening with mammography. He goes on to state, "Experts at the National Cancer Institute have been cautious. The Institute has issued a statement that there is 'suggestive evidence, but no solid proof that mammography benefits now outweigh the risks.'"

He feels, "if you decide to participate, you run a substantial risk of undergoing unnecessary surgery, emotional trauma, and a small, but unknown, risk of possible radiation effects."

"There are insufficient data to indicate that screening for colorectal cancer by stool occult blood testing reduces mortality from the disease in a screened population participating in clinical trials." He doesn't think there is any reason at the time of his book to have a routine stool guaiac test.

As far as routine tests for glaucoma, "Treatment of either elevated intraocular pressure or established glaucoma with conventional drugs has not been shown to produce clear-cut improvement; nor has early treatment been shown to halt the progression of glaucoma. Screening by tonometry is therefore of dubious value."

"Health care intervention produces a preoccupation with disease that detracts from the quality of life and is itself unhealthy ... Most people are fundamentally healthy for most of their lives."

He discusses the many attempts at cost containment and states, "A decrease in medical costs will not automatically insure the best possible medical care. Protecting the quality of care should be a prime consideration in any planning. This consideration has been largely overlooked."

On page 167 Dr. Robin goes through explicit questions which you should ask. He suggests that everyone keep a list of those questions when you go to see your physician.

He comes to a number of conclusions which include reducing the surplus of physicians, reforming the training of medical students, expanding clinical trials, performing only specifically relevant diagnostic procedures, setting more rigorous criteria for screening of normal subjects, assuring adequate support for basic medical science, reducing the number of doctors and hospitals.

He concludes that "10% of the funds now expended each year on unnecessary or harmful medical care would be more than enough to support these suggestions."

Rogatz, Peter. "Let's Get Rid of Those Surplus Hospital Beds." *Prism* (October 1974): 13–4.

Dr. Rogatz states that we need to get rid of surplus hospital beds. Note this was almost two decades ago!

Rosen, Max. *Journal of Urology* (May 1991).

This article indicated that 15% of men who have smoked a pack a day for five years have impotence, 31% who have smoked one pack a day for ten years, and 60% who have smoked one pack a day for 20 years.

Sadusk, Joseph F., and Lewis C. Robbins. "Proposal for Health-Hazard Appraisal in Comprehensive Health Care." *JAMA* 203:13 (25 March 1968,): 106–10.

Risks are listed as the following within 10 years among 100,000 white women age 40: 351 will develop carcinoma of the breasts if they have not had children; 594 will have artereosclerotic heart disease if they smoke two packs per day and are sedentary; 300 will develop some type of stroke even if they have normal blood pressure but are overweight by 20%; 54 will develop carcinoma of the uterus if they have not had children; 13 will develop rheumatic heart disease even though they have nothing wrong on history and physical findings; 133 will develop cirrhosis of the liver, presumably most of them will be alcoholics; 218 will develop carcinoma of the colon/rectum if they had a father who died of cancer of the colon; 93 will have major motor vehicle accidents; 91 will commit suicide; 210 will develop cancer of the lung from smoking; 72 will have pneumonia; 74 will have high blood pressure with the risks increased by hypertension, diabetes, and excess weight; and 80 will have diabetes if they are 20% overweight. All of those are factors which increase the risks of disease.

Scheier, Ronni. "Who Lives? Who Dies? Who Decides?" *American Medical News* (7 January 1991): 3–4.

The entire issue is devoted to the whole concept of dying, from euthanasia to maintaining life in those who are totally vegetative.

Schleifer, Steven J., et. al. "Lymphocyte Function in Major Depressive Disorder." *Archives of General Psychiatry* 41 (May 1984): 484–6.

In depressed patients there is an absolute decrease in the number of both T and B lymphocytes and lymphocyte stimulation by phyto-hemagglutinin, and other agents are significantly lower than in matched controls.

Schwartz, Harry. "Universal Insurance Won't Cure Infant Mortality." *American Medical News* (20 April 1990): 25.

"It's open season on doctors, as usual."

Infant mortality actually is the lowest in the nation's history and is less than half what it was 25 years ago. One of the biggest problems is that a huge percentage of pregnancies today occur in teenagers.

Despite the fact that in the Soviet Union they have had national medical insurance for more than 70 years, they have more than twice as many infant deaths per live birth as does the United States. The problem is not lack of insurance. The problem is the social situation that allows crack, alcohol, drugs, syphilis, gonorrhea, chlamydia, and teenage pregnancy to be so prevalent in the US..

Sehnert, Keith W. *How to Be Your Own Doctor—Sometimes.* New York: Grosset and Dunlap, 1975.

One of the best helps for knowing when to see a physician. It also offers good self-care advice for many problems for which you do not need to see a physician.

Siemonsma, Harry. "Becoming Well is Up to You." *Healthy Advice* (Pacific Mutual publication) (May/June 1988) 1–3.

The author states, "Sixty percent of all illnesses stems from our life-styles."

We must remember that other people think it's up to 80%.

"Sleep Duration is Linked to Life Span." *Medical World News* (5 March 1979): 30, 32.

This involves a followup of 98.4% of more than 800,000 people followed for 20 years. The mortality rate among men who slept less than four hours a night was 2.8 times higher, and among women 1.5 times higher. On the other hand, men and women who slept more than ten hours had 1.8 times the death rate of those with normal sleep duration.

Sokolsky, Anita. "Bad Faith Expanded to Health Care—A National Perspective." *The Health Lawyer* 3:2 (Fall 1987): 6–8, 28–31.

"There is a growing conflict between a patient's protection versus an insurance company's ability to include an arbitration provision in its health care plan."

The author concludes that the states uniformly disregard arbitration clauses in medical malpractice plans, and she considers this to be "unconscionable and demonstrates bad faith."

Such denial of arbitration "will prove costly to insurers, physicians, and consumers."

Somerville, Janice. "Blues Plan Failure Staggers West Virginia: Liquidation Leaves Dispute Over Bill Payment." *American Medical News* (2 November 1990): 1, 27.

The first Blues plan ever liquidated is discussed in the state of West Virginia. When they went bankrupt, they left $30 million in unpaid bills and 270,000 subscribers without insurance.

Southern Medical Journal (19 November 1991).

Starting in October, the Medicare Hassle Factor will be going into high gear as the entire Medicare program gets a major overhaul. The changes are profound ... affecting fees, coding, procedures, and penalties.

Stearn, Martha. "Medicare: Diagnosis Grim, Prognosis Grimmer." (A newspaper article brought in by a patient. The exact source is unknown, but it looks like something from *The Wall Street Journal*.)

"But I am frightened, for myself and my patients. Our future is grim. I do not have the solution."

Stepney, R. "The Psychology and Pharmacology of Smoking." *International Medicine* 4:3 (1984): 42–5.

Nicotine is very similar to acetylcholine. "In the brain it influences levels of adrenaline, dopamine, and many other neurotransmitters."

Because of its relationship to acetylcholine, it is possible to obtain either arousing or sedative effects, depending upon the dose of nicotine and the speed with which it gets into the body.

Individuals who became smokers by the age of 25 had higher levels on both neuroticism and extroversion when they were 16 than those who do not become smokers. .

"Suit for Chelation." *Acres USA.*

"Physician Jim Frackelton reports from Cleveland that recently one of his patients successfully sued his insurance carrier for chelation therapy payment in small claims municipal court, and he suggests that other physicians might want to advise their patients of this option in the event of nonpayment. In addition, if insurance carriers lose such suits, they may be vulnerable to subsequent bad faith suits."

"The Cleveland judge stated: 'Although chelation therapy may not be the *treatment of choice* for atherosclerosis, it appears to be a broadly accepted professional treatment ... It is interesting to note that Defendant, insurance company, would presumably pay for very expensive bypass surgery where there have been approximately 4,000 deaths in 300,000 cases, but has refused to pay for chelation therapy where there have been approximately 20 deaths in 300,000 cases ... The court finds that Plaintiff's chelation therapy was a necessary treatment recommended by a duly licensed physician and that chelation therapy is a broadly accepted treatment of atherosclerosis.'"

Sullivan, Ronald. "Medical Schools Face Cuts in Aid Over Specialists: State Seeks to Train More Family-Care Physicians." *New York Times* (13 March 1979).

In the state of New York, it was stated that it was reported there was a 74% surplus of medical specialists in New York City, which has eight medical schools and the largest collection of teaching hospitals in the world. The state proposed to reduce the state's per diem Medicaid reimbursement rate to teaching hospitals that are training too many surgeons and not enough family physicians.

Interestingly, of course, Blue Cross Blue Shield of greater New York coupled their reimbursement rate to hospitals to the state Medicaid rate.

The article goes on to report that the Department of Health, Education, and Welfare and the State Health Department are all trying to get medical schools and hospitals to produce more family practitioners, but of course medical specialists such as surgeons generate the major share of hospital income.

Taylor, Robert B: "Health Promotion: Can it Succeed in the Office?" *Preventive Medicine* 10 (1981): 258–62.

The conclusion is, "If health promotion is to succeed in the office, if it is to become an integral component of ambulatory health care, then we must reexamine our own thinking as health care providers. The physician must remodel his own personal value system so that he derives personal satisfaction not only from diseases cured and prevented, but also from helping patients achieve optimal health—with less dependence on healers."

I can say that, as far as I can tell, this has not happened in the last ten years since that article was written.

Templin, Neal. "Johnson & Johnson Wellness Plan Shows Healthy Bottom Line." *Wall Street Journal* (Monday, 21 May 1990): 1B, 3B.

It was estimated that companies, just through hospitalization costs, pay an average per employee of $350 per year for smokers; $64 for those with hypertension; and $15 for those with nutritional problems. And 56% of those increased costs due to smoking, high blood pressure, and poor diet are attributed to employees over 54.

The article emphasizes that Johnson & Johnson, one of the largest pharmaceutical and related products companies in the country, was paying $200 per employee to offer check-ups and offer healthier eating and exercise, and that was saving them $378 per employee in medical expenses.

Medical expenses at Johnson & Johnson, which is self-insured, had risen 310% the previous decade.

It is estimated that 30 similar companies had increased costs of 460%. But those increases only minimally went to physicians; most went to hospitals and bureaucracy.

Thomas, Caroline Bedell, and O. Lee McCabe. "Precursors of Premature Disease and Death: Habits of Nervous Tension." *The Johns Hopkins Medical Journal* 147 (1980): 137–45.

Medical students who later developed cancer, coronary occlusion, hypertension, or mental illness, or who committed suicide, were compared with those students who remained healthy 15–30 years later. Habits of nervous tension were significantly greater in people when they were medical students if they were going to develop cancer, coronary occlusion, mental illness, or suicide later in life.

Tolchin, Martin. "Health Care Report Finds Deficiencies." *Columbia Missourian* 67 (2 December 1988): 1.

"More than 4,000 of the nation's 15,000 nursing homes administer drugs without regard to a physician's written orders."

"Nearly 3,000 nursing homes fail to provide rehabilitative nursing care to prevent conditions ranging from immobility to paralysis, and more than 6,500 nursing homes serve food under unsatisfactory conditions."

Toufexis, Anastasia. "Drowsy America." *Time* (17 December 1990): 78–85.

They state that "a typical adult needs about eight hours shut-eye a night to function effectively."

"Perhaps the most insidious consequence of skipping on sleep is the irritability that increasingly pervades society."

"The United States Department of Transportation reports that up to 200,000 traffic accidents each year may be sleep related and about 20% of all drivers have dozed off at least once while behind the wheel."

There is an alarming increase in the frequency of errors made by people who work between 11:00 p.m. and 7:00 a.m. For instance, between 4:00 a.m. and 6:00 a.m. "the rate of fatigue related accidents for single trucks is ten times as high as the rate during the day."

Sleep deprived individuals have problems performing mentally as well as physically.

"About a third of Americans have trouble falling asleep or staying asleep, problems that result in listlessness and loss of alertness during the day."

"U.S. Health Care Facts, Figures Describe a National Catastrophe." *New Sense Bulletin* 16:10 (July 1991): 7.

This article featured the following quotes.

"At least 35 million Americans have no health insurance whatsoever—no policies of their own, no eligibility for public programs."

"Many people are forced to sell their homes to pay medical bills."

"Young adults, followed by children under age 18, are the most likely to be without coverage."

"Insurance provides only limited protection."

"Further, any major claim is likely to cause a phenomenal increase for subsequent coverage—if, in fact, the insurance company deigns to renew the patient."

The reasons existing for what they consider to be the absurd expense of medical care in this country are "inflation; increased numbers of the elderly; more surviving premature infants; increased medical liability; ever more complex billing procedures; the subsidization of the uninsured by the insured; the lack of preventive care; and increased income for doctors." Actually, the latter is *not* true; doctors' income is dropping.

Vaisrub, Samuel. Letter to the editor. *JAMA* 241 (27 April 1979): 1827.

"Clear disjunction between quality and quantity is possible only on a relatively high level of abstraction."

Veatch, Robert M. "Voluntary Risks to Health: The Ethical Issues." *JAMA* 243:1 (4 January 1980): 50–5.

This is one of the few articles which deals with whether or not one should actually "subsidize" public attention to poor health habits.

"Behaviors as highly diverse as smoking, skiing, playing professional football, compulsive eating, omitting exercise, exposing oneself excessively to the sun, skipping needed immunizations, automobile racing, and mountain climbing all can be viewed as having a substantial voluntary component."

Dr. Keith Reemtsma, Chairman of the Department of Surgery at Columbia University, has called for "a more rational approach to improving national health" involving "a reward/punishment system based on individual choices."

He (Dr. Reemtsma) would actually tax people who smoke cigarettes, drink whiskey, drive cars, and own guns. These individuals should be "personally responsible for their health."

He (the author) quotes the first major health hazard appraisal of Belloc and Breslow, which showed that eating moderately, eating regularly, eating breakfast, no cigarette smoking, moderate or no use of alcohol, moderate exercise, and seven to eight hours of sleep lead to a 70-year-old individual having the same average physical health as persons age 35 to 44 who have less than three of those same health habits!

The author argues that even though health and disease are governed by behaviors and risk factors subject to being controlled, society should assume some responsibility for bringing about the changes necessary to produce better health. Part of this argument is based upon the fact that "virtually for every disease, those who are the poorest, those who are in the lowest socioeconomic classes, are at greatest risk."

He tends to side with the fact that "voluntary behaviors are, in reality, the result of social and cultural forces."

Waldman, Steven. "The Insurance Mess." *Newsweek* (23 April 1990): 46–50.

They start by quoting that, in one family, the family spends as much on insurance as the total cost of clothes, heating, bus fare, and day care for their baby.

In 1982 total premiums paid for insurance were $263 billion for automobile insurance, compared with $475 billion in 1989.

Washington State Fund Provider Newsletter (Spring 1987).

It is mentioned that it takes 7 to 14 days "to recover from acute pain associated with joint, ligament and disc sprains or strains."

"Tolerance to narcotics, necessitating increasing doses to achieve the same analgesic effect, occurs at approximately one month."

They mention the fact that even post-operatively it is rare for patients to require strong narcotics beyond the second or third post-operative day.

They state that "the inappropriate prescribing and dispensing of drugs, mainly controlled substances, is the largest single category of disciplinary actions against physicians in Washington and Oregon."

"What's Hot." *Wall Street Journal* (Monday, 13 November 1989): R5.

The fastest-growing procedures, estimated by the Wilkerson Group and Health Care Knowledge Systems.

Outpatient procedures, done in ambulatory surgery centers:

	Average Cost to Patient
ESWL (lithotripsy for breaking up kidney stones)	$10,000

Radioisotope bone scan (used in detecting cancer)	350
Fiberoptic bronchoscopy of lung	
(examines the lung through a fiber optic tube)	350
Diagnostic procedures on fetus and amnion	1,000
MRI (magnetic resonance image)	850
Endoscopy of large bowel	500
Mechanical ventilation (mechanical breather)	
(cost of maintenance and personnel)	300–600
PTCA (coronary angioplasty)	4,000
Cardiac catheterization (left heart) and coronary	
arteriography (usually done at the same time)	3,000

Inpatient hospital procedures:

	Average Cost to Patient
Phototherapy (use of ultraviolet light in treatment of skin conditions and jaundice in infants)	$ 140
MRI	850
ESWL	10,000
PTCA	4,000
Insertion of inflatable penile prosthesis	4,000
Laser angioplasty (treats blood vessel blockage)	8,000
Fiberoptic bronchoscopy of lung	350
Diagnostic procedures on fetus and amnion	1,000
Mechanical ventilation	300-600
Temporary pacemaker	5,000

Will, George F. "The Hot Seat." *Newsweek* (7 March 1977): 96.

The author indicated that "Today nearly 10% of gross national product is spent on medical care."

"General Motors has said that there is more medicine than steel in its automobiles; in this sense: it spends more on health care premiums for employees than it spends on steel."

Wynder, Ernest, L., and Peter Peacock. "The Practice of Disease Prevention." *JAMA* 229:23 (23 September 1974): 1743.

Dr. Ernest L. Wynder and Peter Petercock of the American Health Foundation argue that the problem is one of apathy. They emphasize apathy on the part of the public and among physicians, as physicians are trained to deal with illness.

They point out that in Germany in 1883 it was not called "health insurance," it was called "sickness insurance."

The authors argue that "preventive care" would become "the first line of defense in tomorrow's medical care delivery system."

They state that both physicians and the public have an attitude of disease, "the practice of disease" enhancement.

"We need to recognize that many of today's chronic illnesses have preventable causes."

Zwick, Daniel. "Health Policy Guidelines and Holistic Care." *Journal of Medical Education* 52 (1977): 648–53.

This article lists the purposes, timetable, and processes connected to the development of National Health Policy Guidelines mandated by Public Law 93–641. Six major dimensions were selected by the Department of Health, Education, and Welfare Task Force, which included a unifying theme of wellness with the role of the federal government in defining and implementing national goals and standards including the concept of health enhancement, the concept of wellness health innovation, dealing with new procedures and products entering the health care delivery field, and "health promotion and protection, which will be concerned with health maintenance, prevention, environmental, and related issues."

Needless to say, there is no evidence that this ever went anywhere. We wonder how many millions were spent on that task force.

As early as June 22, 1976, I sent the following note to the International Academy of Preventive Medicine:

"Voluntary self-regulation has been demonstrated over the past 50 years to be the single most effective modality for teaching people 'Health Maintenance.' Every physiological process studied to date has been found to be capable of being brought under voluntary control. The combination of biofeedback, autogenic training, related auto-suggestive type exercise, and a psychosynthesis approach have been combined into a system for presenting this both to patients with a variety of illness and as a health maintenance or preventive approach for normal individuals."

Typical letters from major insurance companies such as Aetna ... "We analyze bills submitted to us by other medical providers in your area for similar services. Your charges exceed area prevailing fees." Interestingly, this seems to happen to *every* physician's office, so where do they get the prevailing fees?

Here is a letter I received from Blue Cross Blue Shield of Minnesota, August 12, 1985.

"Since the cost-effectiveness of your program cannot be bettered by any of the programs currently operating in Minnesota, we are very curious to now ask your opinion of several points ... We are very impressed with the economic incentives associated with an effectively utilized program of comprehensive pain treatment."

In 1989 Blue Cross Blue Shield of St. Louis denied all payments for treatment of a patient whom we saw for agitated depression and low back pain. His depression was the result of his low back pain. He did have some physical mechanical abnormalities in the back. Despite that, Blue Cross Blue Shield refused to pay the fee.

I wrote a letter to the Chief Executive Officer of Blue Cross Blue Shield stating, "This is typical bureaucratic nonsense. I will personally assist this patient in instituting a law suit against you if this is not settled more reasonably. I'm asking the insurance commissioner of the state of Missouri to investigate Blue Cross Blue Shield, not only because of this, but because of all the dawdling that has gone on in your office in the last year and a half. You do not answer my letters, and this is not the first that I have written. I consider your company totally irresponsible, unethical, unprofessional, and the most obnoxious insurance company in this entire country."

As a result of that, I was sent a letter by the president stating, "I am offended by the statements contained in your letter of August 23. Blue Cross Blue Shield has been exceedingly patient in attempting to assist you; that patience is exhausted and we will respond to you only as required by Medicare contract. We are cancelling your participating physician status with Blue Cross and Blue Shield of Missouri effective October 10, 1989. Further, I have referred your letter to the corporate counsel for further consideration."

I have not heard from their counsel or them since then, but it is of considerable interest that sometime shortly thereafter one of their employees reported me to the state medical licensing board claiming apparently that I had falsified some records submitted to them. That was supposed to have been discussed at the state medical board meeting in May 1990, and I have heard nothing from them since that time. If that individual at Blue Cross Blue Shield had proved that we had done something fraudulent, he had many more available tactics that he could have carried out, such as publicly proclaiming that we had done something fraudulently and denying me any participation in Medicare. It appears to me, as far as I can tell, that this was just one of their behind-the-scenes attempts to harass a physician.

In one week I have received three really obnoxious, threatening notices from the Department of Health and Human Services, including such things as a special fraud alert. This particular one states that it is illegal for physicians to waive deductibles or co-payments to Medicare patients. The penalties for doing this can amount to many thousands of dollars.

Here is an indication of the way in which your Medicare intermediaries waste money. The General American Life Insurance Company put on a "Health Insurance Expo 91" September 25–27, 1991, free of charge to physicians celebrating General American's 25 years as Medicare intermediaries. Well, they *should* celebrate because it certainly is where they make a lot of their profit.

They even had a session called "Who says there is no such thing as a free lunch? We'll give you one, buffet style, in the vendor area." They had complimentary beverages and hors d'oeuvres two nights.

It's one of those really pleasant things where they try to make you think they're really a nice group of people, and in my opinion they're among the most obnoxious in the world.

On July 25, 1984, the President of the Greene County Medical Society sent a letter to all Greene County physicians outlining the severe problems with the St. Louis Blue Shield plan in which Blue Cross Blue Shield had started informing its subscribers that they could not be billed for any fees not paid for by Blue Shield to so-called UCR physicians, that those physicians were only supposed to be paid their usual customary and reasonable fee. Suddenly Blue Cross Blue Shield had started *setting* those fees.

The President of the organization outlined some of the problems. "Apparently, payment amounts were not consistent for the same or similar procedures, and in some cases months passed before payment was received. Request for data as to how current levels of reimbursement were computed were delayed, turned aside, or refused."

The President went on to cite a case in the United States District Court of Massachusetts which had rendered a similar problem by the Massachusetts Blue Shield organization as illegal and an unreasonable restraint of trade and an anti-trust violation. The judge found that the policy "would tend to inhibit the introduction and dissemination of new medical techniques and provided no reward for excellence or any incentive qualitative improvement or innovation by physicians."

Thus, the Society recommended that we withdraw as UCR participants, and I submitted by resignation to Blue Shield of St. Louis on May 22, 1984.

A memo sent to Missouri surgeons from the Missouri State Surgical Society.

This memo "calls for immediate action" to all Missouri surgeons.

"Despite assurance that the new system of RBRVS would be budget neutral, the proposed rule contains a drastic 16% reduction in the initial conversion factor."

And they of course are urging us to try to get Congress to intervene—As if Congress ever improves anything.

According to an update from St. Paul Professional Malpractice Division, nearly 70% of the failures to diagnose cancer claims cite the physician's office or clinic as having committed malpractice because of failure to diagnose cancer, but surgical issues still dominate the highest number of claims, representing 28.8% of all malpractice claims.

THE LOST PYRAMIDS OF ROCK LAKE
BY FRANK JOSEPH

Was Atlantis in Wisconsin? Now, for the first time, here is proof of ancient, sacred pyramids at the bottom of a small lake in Wisconsin! Learn about the fascinating secrets of a great people who erected structures on land and in water as sophisticated astronomical observatories for their bloody sky cult.

This lake is 40 miles west of Milwaukee, Wisconsin. In 1989 author Frank Joseph organized the first side-scan sonar sweep of Rock Lake for the elusive structures. His instruments revealed an unprecedented panorama on the lake floor by way of images transposed from sound waves. The high-tech method identified a colossal stone mound shaped like an elongated pyramid 60 feet below the surface, and his research subsequently received widespread attention in the regional press.

Joseph has traveled the world over for revealing clues to the lost history of prehistoric Wisconsin, and is presently working with state authorities to have Rock Lake declared an official historic site. Trace the development of this ancient culture and read about amazing parallels with similar prehistoric cultures in the Canary Islands.

1-880090-04-X, 6 x 9, 220 pgs., illus., softbound $10.95

JOURNEYS: The Adventures of Leaf
BY LOUANN CARROLL

Journeys is a delightful story for young and old readers alike. It is the tale of a distressed maple leaf whose tenuous hold on the tree is broken by the cool, fall wind. His many adventures teach him much about life and friendship. He believes his life is over, but when we read about a new bud on the same tree in the following springtime, we know the spirit of Leaf has been reborn in a new form.

Included are delightful drawings from a seventh-grade art class who had listened to the story, demonstrating the impact the story's values had on the insightful students. These drawings are suitable for coloring in a variety of mediums.

Although this is a children's story, each person who reads *Journeys* interprets it differently. To the author it means:

"Life is full of journeys. Some roads you choose are more difficult than others. Though some people would believe you are wrong in your choosing, each person is guided by their inner being to that choice which is right for them. You must not feel guilty that your choice sometimes differs from what is thought best by those who love you. You must live your life, then die, only to live again."

1-880090-03-1, 10 x 8, 60 pgs., illus.   **$9.95**

HOLY ICE: Bridge to the Subconscious
BY FRANK DORLAND

Holy Ice is a unique book about crystals—not any crystals, but real *electronic quartz crystal*. Electronic crystal is that flawlesss form of crystal which is used in countless electrical components. Most naturally occurring quartz crystal is not electronic. Only a small percentage of high quality material (absolutely clear) will perform. It is the high quality crystal that was mankind's first solid-state device.

A live, electronic crystal was born many years ago deep in the Earth from the forces of fire and water. The ancients called it "Holy Ice," and said it was frozen holy water spilled out of heaven.

In ancient times, the crystals were shaped by craftsmen into working crystals which resembled semi-round balls and talismanic symbols such as moons, crosses and the like. These working crystals were in daily use for healing purposes as well as for protection and survival.

Mr. Dorland has taken ancient information about the use of quartz crystal and made it accessible for modern-day understanding and practical usage. He clearly explains how the subconscious acts and how to reprogram behavior and thinking using crystals for successful and peaceful living.

1-880090-02-3, 6 x 9, 192 pgs., illus., color plates $12.95

HUMOR TRAVELS WELL
BY PETE DOCHERTY

A funny story can happen anywhere, and here is a book that proves it. Written by Peter Docherty, the president of a travel incentive business in Edina, Minnesota, *Humor Travels Well* is a collection of 22 heartwarming and hilarious stories taken from the author's experiences as a travel professional.

With this book, you'll travel with Pete to places and situations beyond imagination—to lunching with nobility, being detained at a Soviet airport and attending a third-rate English theatre (where you'll witness theatrics with a drama all their own). You'll discover how Pete learned the subtleties of Brazilian sign language, how he summoned up enough politeness to eat a sheep's eyeball, and how he managed to keep his cool as an honored guest at a human cremation.

But best of all, the stories in *Humor Travels Well* will introduce you to unforgettable people from around the world. You'll meet celebrities and royalty from many nations, serious as well as drunken officials, snake charmers and maharajahs, students of many specialities—from medicine to American slang—not to mention the American travelers for whom Pete has served as a guide.

And you'll find that humor is truly the universal language—from Beijing to Barbados, Rome to Rio, the Soviet Union to Scandinavia. Let Pete Docherty be your guide to adventures of all kinds across the globe. We guarantee that you won't need a translator!

1-880090-00-7, 5-1/4 x 8, 192 pgs., illus.   **$5.95**

ESSENCE OF RELIGION
BY ALLISON L. BAYLES

A delightful book about the common spirituality of all the world's greatest religions. Focusing on what unites rather than separates us, this primer is devoted to a better understanding of God and the works of His many hands, which inspire to awe and humility. It is dedicated to all people who yearn to find a way to have life and to have it more abundantly, with blessed assurance.

After concluding that religion is an indispensable element in life, Allison Bayles examines the Seven Great Religions. His choice is Episcopalian, but he retains a profound love and sympathetic understanding of each religion. They all have common elements, such as the Golden Rule and the existence of God. The essay ends with a discussion of Gandhi's seven social sins.

This unique primer requires only an hour to read. There is no attempt to proselytize, but rather to help you understand and appreciate the religion to which you have been exposed, and your relationship to the world community and the Universe.

1-880090-08-2, 4-1/4 x 51/2, 80 pgs. **$5.95**

To order books, please send full amount plus $2.00 for postage and handling for orders under $10.00.
For order over $10.00, please include $3.00 s/h.

Send orders to:

Galde Press, Inc.
PO Box 65611-T
St. Paul MN 55165